→ Doing ←

MENTAL HEALTH
RESEARCH
with CHILDREN
and ADOLESCENTS

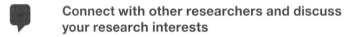
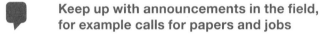
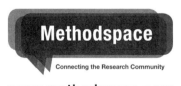
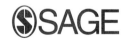

Doing
MENTAL HEALTH
RESEARCH
with CHILDREN
and ADOLESCENTS

A Guide to Qualitative Methods

by
MICHELLE O'REILLY
and NICOLA PARKER

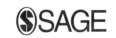

Los Angeles | London | New Delhi
Singapore | Washington DC

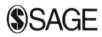

Los Angeles | London | New Delhi
Singapore | Washington DC

SAGE Publications Ltd
1 Oliver's Yard
55 City Road
London EC1Y 1SP

SAGE Publications Inc.
2455 Teller Road
Thousand Oaks, California 91320

SAGE Publications India Pvt Ltd
B 1/I 1 Mohan Cooperative Industrial Area
Mathura Road
New Delhi 110 044

SAGE Publications Asia-Pacific Pte Ltd
3 Church Street
#10-04 Samsung Hub
Singapore 049483

Editor: Kate Wharton
Assistant editor: Laura Walmsley
Production editor: Rachel Burrows
Copyeditor: Helen Skelton
Proofreader: Anna Gilding
Indexer: Martin Hargreaves
Marketing manager: Camille Richmond
Cover design: Lisa Harper-Wells
Typeset by: C&M Digitals (P) Ltd, Chennai, India
Printed in India at Replika Press Pvt Ltd

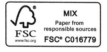

At SAGE we take sustainability seriously. Most of our
products are printed in the UK using FSC papers and
boards. When we print overseas we ensure sustainable
papers are used as measured by the Egmont
grading system. We undertake an annual audit to
monitor our sustainability.

Library of Congress Control Number: 2014930360

British Library Cataloguing in Publication data

A catalogue record for this book is available from
the British Library

ISBN 978-1-4462-7070-7
ISBN 978-1-4462-7071-4 (pbk)

CONTENTS

LIST OF FIGURES AND TABLES

Figures

Tables

ABOUT THE AUTHORS

Dr Michelle O'Reilly is a Senior Lecturer at the University of Leicester, for the Greenwood Institute of Child Health. Michelle has an interest in various areas of child mental health, undertaking research in autism, self-harm, family therapy and mental health assessments. She favours the methods of discourse and conversation analysis. Michelle is the director of two language-based research groups. The Language and Interaction Research Assembly (LIRA) is a University of Leicester interdisciplinary group who utilise a range of qualitative language-based approaches. Conversation Analysis Research in Autism (CARA) is an international group who utilise discourse and conversation analytic approaches in the study of autism. Michelle has recently published two books: *Research with Children: Theory and Practice* (Sage) and *A Practical Guide to Mental Health Problems in Children with Autistic Spectrum Disorder* (JKP).

Dr Nicola Parker is a Senior Clinical Psychologist currently working for the Cheshire and Wirral Partnership NHS Foundation Trust. She has clinical experience in the assessment and implementation of therapeutic interventions with children and families, particularly those in Looked After settings including foster care and adoptive families. Nicola also has a wealth of practical experience working with children and young people for more than two decades as a Youth Worker, School Governor, Business Mentor and Prison Volunteer. In addition she has worked for Relate UK and Samaritans as a project manager developing curriculum for children and training counsellors in working with young people. Before embarking on a Clinical career, Nicola completed a PhD in Psychology to further her research interest in the interactions between adults and children in therapeutic settings. Her research is informed by a social constructionist perspective favouring the analysis of intergenerational interactions in therapy environments using discursive approaches.

PREFACE

This book is an introductory text to illustrate the key issues faced when undertaking a child mental health research project. It provides an accessible guide through each element of the research process from inception to dissemination/application. It is designed to help students, trainees, researchers, academics and others in health, mental health, social care, education, or other disciplines to plan and undertake a qualitative project. This is a timely text given the growing emphasis within mental health services on evidence-based practice.

The focus of this book is on doing research *with* rather than *about* children, which is congruent with the contemporary perspective of giving children their own 'voice' through research. Nonetheless, the importance of doing research with significant adults, including parents and professionals involved in caring for or working with children with mental health difficulties, is considered alongside this. The need for systematic and practical advice for researchers has dictated the focus of each chapter; each of which is filled with helpful tips and advice.

Definitions

Throughout the book a number of concepts/terms are employed. To assist you we outline the ways in which these are utilised. For example, where the pronoun 'we' is used, we refer to the authors and the pronoun 'you' refers to the reader.

As this book focuses on child mental health research, we recognise the importance of defining the way in which we use the term 'mental health'. The definition utilised by the World Health Organization (WHO) which is most widely accepted defines mental health as:

> ... a state of well-being in which every individual realizes his or her own potential, can cope with the normal stresses of life, can work productively and fruitfully, and is able to make a contribution to her or his community. (WHO, 2011: 1)

Whilst this applies to mental health in all populations, for children there are some additional specific indicators related to chronological and developmental age. One widely cited definition of child mental health is offered by the Mental Health Foundation (1999) and is used here as a benchmark against which mental health and mental health difficulties are demarcated in this book. The key elements are: to develop psychologically, creatively, spiritually, emotionally and intellectually; to initiate, develop and sustain personal relationships; to enjoy and use solitude; to be aware of others and express empathy; to learn and play; to develop a sense of right and wrong; and to be able to resolve problems and setbacks and learn from them.

We acknowledge there are a range of different terms used when referring to the absence of positive mental health, including mental illness, mental disorder, mental health problem, mental health difficulty, mental health conditions and mental ill health. Each of these terms tend to be under-pinned by different models which dictate the terms favoured, for example, the medical profession may prefer terminology such as 'illness'. For the purpose of clarity and consistency in relation to conducting research we employ the general term 'mental health difficulty'.

Unless otherwise specified, we use the term 'child/children' throughout the book as an overarching category which encompasses children of all ages from 0–18 years. Where it is required to differentiate age groups we employ the categories of 'younger child', 'young child' and 'older child' to distinguish chronological age groups, 0–4 years, 5–11 years and 12–18 years respectively.

The term 'parent/parents' is used throughout the book to refer to all adults who have legal responsibility for children, this includes foster parents, adoptive parents, biological parents, step-parents, carers, legal guardians and local authorities.

ACKNOWLEDGEMENTS

We would like to offer our appreciation to several people who have helped to make this book happen. Nadzeya Svirydzenka made an important contribution to the information on transcription by translating Russian data into English and contributed to the interview in the chapter on dissemination. Panos Vostanis also contributed to the transcription detail by translating data into Greek and provided useful comments for the research setting chapter by discussing his work with homeless children. We are very grateful for their time. Nisha Dogra contributed to the interview for the dissemination chapter, discussing the challenges relevant to disseminating to children and we thank her for these insights. Tom Muskett and Jessica Lester also contributed interviews for the book. Tom made a useful contribution in discussing the challenges of occupying dual roles and Jessica talked about her experiences of being reflexive in the research process. We very much appreciate these important discussions. We also thank Victoria Stafford for sharing her insights in conducting pilot studies and offering practical comments on this aspect of the chapter on planning. We thank Arthritis Research UK and Elizabeth Hale for allowing us to copy their press release in the dissemination chapter as this is an especially useful example of this form of dissemination. We want to extend our appreciation and give special thanks to Khalid Karim and Claire Bone for their useful and insightful comments on the book as a whole as we feel that the book is much improved because of it. We also thank the two anonymous reviewers for their suggestions to develop areas within the book and all of their ideas. Of course we thank our partners and families for their personal support during the process of writing, for their patience and understanding. Finally we thank SAGE, for facilitating this book from inception to publication.

LIST OF ABBREVIATIONS

CA	Conversation analysis
CAMHS	Child and Adolescent Mental Health Services
CBT	Cognitive behaviour therapy
CRB	Criminal Records Bureau (now referred to as DBS – see below)
DA	Discourse analysis
DBS	Disclosure and Barring Service
DP	Discursive psychology
GP	General Practitioner
IPA	Interpretative phenomenological analysis
OCD	Obsessive compulsive disorder
RCT	Randomised controlled trial
SRA	Social Research Association
UK	United Kingdom
WHO	World Health Organization

PART ONE
THEORY AND BACKGROUND

CHAPTER 1

THEORY AND UTILITY OF QUALITATIVE RESEARCH

Learning outcomes

- Distinguish between audit, service evaluation and research.
- Differentiate between quantitative and qualitative research with children.
- Recognise and appreciate the position of different theories in research.
- Appreciate the differences between methodologies and methods.

Introduction

This chapter opens by distinguishing research projects from audits and service evaluations. These distinctions are important as they have implications for ethics and practical decisions regarding the purpose of the study. This is followed by an introduction to the distinctions between methodological approaches. To enable informed decisions about how to proceed with your research we start by explaining the differences between quantitative and qualitative research with children. Research aims to generate new knowledge or test something that is already known. We explore different theories about how knowledge is generated and how adherence to different theoretical perspectives will impact on the choices you make when planning your project. Discussions of theory and the terminology around these concepts may feel quite daunting to the new researcher. In this chapter we take a step-by-step approach to explain what these terms mean and why they are important.

Audit, service evaluation and research

Before you start your child mental health project you need to be certain that you are planning to do research, not an audit or service evaluation. See Table 1.1.

Table 1.1   Audit, service evaluation and research

Type	Description
Audit	Refers to a process of measuring current practices against a predefined set of standards. It compares practice with best practice (Closs & Cheater, 1996).
Service evaluation	Refers to the evaluation of service provision with a view to setting objectives for improvement. It seeks to assess the effectiveness of interventions to determine whether they met their objectives (Nolan & Grant, 1993).
Research	Refers to a process of establishing knowledge which forms an evidence-base for good practice. It tends to be driven by theory and should relate to broader populations/settings (Black, 1992).

The main difference between these is their purpose. Service evaluations and audits tend to be concerned with monitoring and assessing whether predefined standards are being met and setting service goals. Research is concerned with generating knowledge and understanding phenomena.

 If you have established your project as research not audit, it is important you conform to the standards required.

Differentiating qualitative and quantitative research with children

Although the focus of this book is specifically qualitative research it is useful to understand some of its differences from quantitative approaches. In simple terms quantitative research is concerned with measuring 'quantity' and qualitative research is concerned with the 'quality' of individual experiences.

Quantitative research with children

The aim of quantitative research is to generate large-scale numerical data to predict trends. Typically quantitative research takes a 'scientific' approach to ensure a replicable and robust piece of research, often testing cause and effect or the relationships between variables. Quantitative approaches start with hypotheses, which are predictions of what is expected to happen; these are then tested to see if those predictions are correct and if so whether generalisations can be made.

Example

A researcher may predict (hypothesise) that clinically obese children experience lower self-esteem than other children. A quantitative research project might be designed to measure self-esteem in this cohort and compare that with children within a healthy BMI range. The results may be expected to be the same (generalisable) in the wider child population.

Qualitative research with children

The aim of qualitative research is to explore the individual experiences, beliefs and perceptions of children. Usually qualitative research is conducted with smaller numbers and is concerned with examining depth rather than breadth. Qualitative research starts with an open question, such as *'what'*, *'how'*, *'why'*, or *'when'* to investigate what an issue means to children. The process in qualitative designs is as important as the outcomes.

Example

A qualitative researcher is interested in the relationship between obesity and self-esteem in children and designs a study to explore children's experiences of their weight and their self-esteem. The findings take the form of looking at patterns in the words that children use to talk about their experiences. These findings can help researchers understand children's thoughts and feelings on this issue and may give an indication of how other children in the same situation might feel (transferability).

In health there has been a growth of qualitative research and greater calls to include qualitative findings in supporting evidence-based practice (Sandelowski, 2004).

Illuminating the differences

We outline the distinctions between these two approaches in Table 1.2.

Table 1.2   Differences

Quantitative	Qualitative
Makes predictions about children and their behaviour and then tests those predictions.	Starts with an open question about a child related topic and then explores it.
Considered an objective approach.	Considered a subjective approach.
Tries to reduce any impact that the researcher may have during the process.	Accepts that the researcher will inevitably influence the research process.
Makes generalisations from the results about other children in the same situation.	The findings can be used to help understand other children in similar situations.
Uses statistics to analyse the data.	Analyses children's words or texts.
Interested in cause/effect or relationships between things.	Interested in how children make sense of things.
Focuses mostly on outcomes.	Focuses mostly on process.

These broad differences are widely accepted and may be helpful to you in deciding which one you prefer. The table presented may seem to suggest that your choice is either/or, but in some cases researchers may choose to design their research project in two phases, incorporating both a quantitative and qualitative element. This is known as mixed-methods research design.

Example

Phase one (quantitative) may be to ascertain the number of children who are clinically obese and also have low self-esteem. This will indicate the frequency or the extent of the problem. Phase two (qualitative) may be to explore how these children experience feelings of poor self-image.

Although it may appear that quantitative and qualitative research are quite separate, viewing the two approaches as dichotomous may oversimplify the issue and it may be more useful to think of all methods as on a spectrum (Peters, 2010).

Case example: The value of a qualitative approach in child mental health research

Rajesh is a paediatrician carrying out his research on refugee children's experiences of anxiety. Rajesh found that these children are particularly anxious when visiting his clinics and he is interested in the reasons why; he thinks it may be related to discrimination and stigma. He is currently attempting to write down his ideas to show his colleagues and is struggling to decide which approach would be most suitable.

A   **Activity   Case example**

Consider in what ways a qualitative methodology might be most appropriate to explore this topic. Reflect on the assumptions Rajesh is making and how this might influence his research.

You may have considered a range of different reasons why a qualitative approach is suitable. This might include the main purpose of his study being to explore children's accounts of their own subjective experiences as refugees. He is clearly interested in ascertaining personal reports of anxiety rather than clinical scales or measurements. The qualitative approach provides an opportunity to discover aspects of their experiences that may not have been anticipated by Rajesh.

It would be beneficial through supervision for Rajesh to reflect on his assumptions about these children experiencing discrimination in their host country. It is possible that not all of the children experience discrimination, or may not be aware of discriminatory behaviour against them. Furthermore Rajesh is assuming that any anxiety experienced by these children is caused by discrimination/stigma rather than considering that it may be attributed to a complex interplay of other factors.

The role of theory

From the literature you are likely to come across specific terminology that researchers use. Although it might be tempting to skip over these, the concepts they represent are important to help inform your choices. There are five key concepts that we briefly consider here: *paradigm, ontology, epistemology, methodology* and *methods*, illustrated in Figure 1.1. We advise you to consult other texts for additional information, for example, Pascale (2011).

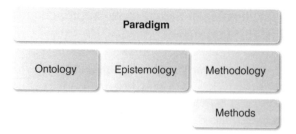

Figure 1.1   Concepts and theory

Paradigm – a set of beliefs and practices that define a particular discipline

Thomas Kuhn (1962) is often credited as being one of the original writers on the issue of scientific paradigms, arguing that paradigms refer to a set of practices that define a particular scientific discipline at a given period of time. Kuhn argued that paradigms are scientific achievements providing model problems and solutions for communities of researchers. A paradigm in social and health research therefore is viewed as a basic set of beliefs representing a particular worldview, which includes specific beliefs and meanings. Paradigms constitute an overarching framework for understanding how the world operates and provide structure for the direction research should take and how it should be performed.

Ontology – the nature of reality and what can be known about it

Ontologies are theories about the nature of existence and address the question of what can be known (Pascale, 2011). Ontology deals with questions in relation to what can exist or what is said to exist. It is important to recognise that ontological questions are fundamental in research as they constitute the foundations of social inquiry (Pascale, 2011). The three most common ontological positions which most researchers align with are realism, critical realism and relativism (Guba & Lincoln, 2004).

First is realism. The researcher believes in an objective reality that can be uncovered through research and which is contrasted with a subjective reality. An objective reality means that there is a reality that is outside an individual's interpretations or imagination. This objective external world can be represented through language, thoughts, beliefs and desires, as well as physical artefacts such as pictures and maps (Cromby and Nightingale, 1999). Realism believes that this world exists regardless of how we represent it.

> **Example**
>
> A realist researcher undertaking research involving children with ADHD will start from the premise that ADHD exists objectively as a condition which can be measured and understood through research.

Second is critical realism. The researcher believes in an objective reality but recognises that personal, social, cultural and historical factors, such as race, gender and economics, subjectively influence the way that reality is understood and experienced. The notion of critical realism has been associated with several schools of thought with slightly different philosophical understandings of the term.

> **Example**
>
> A critical realist researcher undertaking research related to children with ADHD will start from the premise that ADHD exists but will also take into account the ways in which it is constructed and understood within social, political and cultural contexts.

Third is relativism. This stands in opposition to realism and this is often negotiated rhetorically (Edwards et al., 1995). For relativism the researcher believes that there is no objective reality but that all that is 'known' is the product of socially constructed ways of making sense of things. It argues that any external world is actually inaccessible to us in practice and in principle and need not be considered (Cromby & Nightingale, 1999).

> **Example**
>
> A relativist researcher undertaking research related to children with ADHD will start from the premise that ADHD does not exist objectively, but is a contemporary label which has been agreed upon and given meaning only through its social context.

Epistemology – the relationship between the knower, what can be known and how

Epistemology, like ontology, is a branch of philosophy. Epistemology asks questions regarding how we can know what we know (Pascale, 2011) and is concerned with the nature and scope of knowledge. Epistemology can be understood as a 'justificatory account' of the production of scientific knowledge (Pascale, 2011). Although there are many (and some contention regarding what constitutes epistemologies), three common epistemological positions are positivism, post-positivism and social constructionism.

Positivism assumes that knowledge about the world is derived from objective facts and draws upon the principles of the natural sciences to make its claims. It is based on the idea that information which is logical, scientific and mathematical is the most valid knowledge. Positivist researchers believe that aspects of humanity can be measured objectively.

Example

A positivist researcher interested in investigating autism would start from the premise that knowledge about what constitutes autism can be gained through objective measures, usually quantitative. Positivists believe that autism exists independently and its symptoms can be measured to determine whether or not it is present in the child.

Post-positivism recognises that evidence in research is always imperfect. This position identifies that socio-political factors influence the way knowledge is shaped (Robson, 2011). In other words the researcher accepts that their knowledge, values and background may influence what they observe, but still pursues objectivity by recognising and seeking to eliminate this bias. Methods, therefore, should reflect this concern by aiming to reduce bias and seek to describe causal relationships.

Example

A post-positivist researcher interested in investigating autism would also start from the premise that knowledge about what constitutes autism can be measured. However, they would be concerned to remove contextual factors such as social or cultural, which could bias the research results.

Social constructionism is an epistemological position which assumes that knowledge does not pre-exist as a fact which can be discovered, but rather is co-created in a social, historical and political context and cannot be separated from this. In other words this argument advocates that meaning is co-created in and through language and interaction. Thus, research does not aim to discover 'facts' but to look to a more pragmatic and political goal, not searching for the truth, but meaning and experience (Burr, 1995). This means that the social construction of reality is a dynamic process which is reproduced by people and that reality is constructed rather than objective.

Example

A social constructionist researcher interested in investigating autism argues that it can only be understood within the context of an individual's idiosyncratic ways of making sense of their symptoms, the meanings they themselves construct. Autism exists only because people have agreed it does and consolidated its meaning through talk and text.

Methodology – the guiding theories that dictate which methods will be used to acquire knowledge

It is helpful to remember that methodology and methods are different. Methodologies are the 'logical frameworks of research design' while methods are the techniques for acquiring data (Pascale, 2011: 2). In other words, methodology is a design process for carrying out research and methods are the set of tools/instruments to carry out the research. The usefulness of the chosen method will be dependent upon its congruence with the associated ontology, epistemology and methodology.

Example

A researcher interested in Asian girls' experiences of their eating disorders is likely to choose a qualitative methodology and may opt for the data collection method of interviewing with the analytic method of thematic analysis.

This is particularly important in child mental health research which historically has been predominantly quantitative, because positivism resonates with medical practice training where the natural sciences dominate (Peters, 2010). Although this can be useful it is not always appropriate. Qualitative methods for investigating areas of mental health can be especially informative. These methods can help stimulate new ideas and build theories around mental health. The rich data gathered can also be especially helpful in providing terminology which is meaningful to service users and these can be incorporated into clinical practice (Peters, 2010).

> ## *A*   Activity   Building a glossary
>
> We have introduced you to some unfamiliar terms and it may be useful to consolidate your understanding of them by building your own glossary of concepts in your own words.

Summary

This chapter has introduced you to some important concepts associated with research projects in child mental health. You should now be able to distinguish between audit, service evaluation and research. You should be clear regarding the distinction between quantitative and qualitative research and the rationale for using a qualitative approach for your child mental health project. Hopefully you will also be starting to appreciate how your worldview and theoretical position will inform your methodological choices. This in turn will greatly assist you in making decisions about the methods you will use both for data collection and analysis. This chapter provides a foundation for working through the rest of this book.

Key messages

- Audit, research and service evaluation have a different purpose, different aims and objectives and are conducted in different ways.
- Qualitative research aims to explore people's perceptions, experiences, opinions and accounts.
- Quantitative research aims to establish cause and effect or relationships in an objective manner.
- Research is underpinned by particular assumptions about how the world works and methodological choices should be congruent with this worldview.

Further reading

Guba, E. G. & Lincoln, Y. S. (2004). Competing paradigms in qualitative research: Theories and issues. In S. N. Hesse-Biber & P. Leavy (eds), *Approaches to qualitative research: A reader on theory and practice* (pp. 17–38). Oxford: Oxford University Press.

Nightingale, D. & Cromby, J. (eds) (1999). *Social constructionist psychology: A critical analysis of theory and practice*. Buckingham: Open University Press.

Pascale, C-M. (2011). *Cartographies of knowledge: Exploring qualitative epistemologies*. Thousand Oaks, CA: Sage.

CHAPTER 2

THE NEED FOR QUALITATIVE EVIDENCE

Learning outcomes

- Recognise the relationship between clinical practice and research evidence.
- Perform a literature review.
- Critically appraise the evidence.
- Recognise the quality markers.

Introduction

In health, the evidence yielded from research informs interventions, understanding client's experiences and improving communication practices. In this chapter we consider the backdrop of evidence-based practice in child mental health to provide an appreciation of how research evidence fits into the overall political, practical and social framework. To contextualise the value of qualitative evidence we illustrate some of the limitations of relying on controlled trials in child mental health disciplines and illuminate some benefits of including evidence from qualitative work. To appreciate the evidence-base researchers need to be able to conduct literature searches and we provide practical guidance regarding how to do this. Additionally it is important that readers take a critical perspective on the evidence produced and we provide a toolkit for critical reading of journal articles. We conclude the chapter by guiding readers on how to recognise the quality indicators for qualitative research.

The importance of doing child mental health research

One in six adults experience symptoms of mental illness costing the UK £77 billion per year (Stratton, 2010), with approximately 10% of all children in the UK suffering from mental health difficulties at any time and up to 20% in any given year (Halliwell et al., 2007). On the basis of this statistical evidence and the rising costs of supporting children and their families, it may seem obvious that child mental health is a serious problem for services.

However, in child mental health there is a high level of unmet service need (Waddell & Godderis, 2005), which suggests that there is increased need for research to understand the reasons and improve service provision. For this to be effective it is important that high-quality studies are conducted, that researchers disseminate their findings clearly and that practicing professionals draw upon this evidence in their daily work (Rishel, 2007).

Healthcare therefore demands the development of research methods which are robust enough to inform clinical practice, but this can be challenging given the competing methodological frameworks and differing theories (Roy-Chowdhury, 2003). Nonetheless there is increasing pressure to ensure that each area of healthcare has an evidence-base and this means that professionals are facing increasing challenges in their work. This is also true of other professional disciplines such as education and social care.

The relationship between practice and research

Evidence-based practice means that professionals seek to apply knowledge gained from research to improve their work. Originally the concept emerged in the discipline of medicine but other areas have now followed (Waddell & Godderis, 2005). In child mental health the reliance on evidence to inform commissioning decisions is typically used to differentiate the cost-effectiveness and value of various therapeutic modalities and strategies (Hoagwood et al., 2001).

Over time there has been investment in the infrastructure of healthcare to increase the likelihood of interventions being delivered on the basis of best-evidence (Rycroft-Malone et al., 2004). The importance of evidence-based practice resonates with credibility and enables professionals to modify their practice (Small, 2005). This means that the concept of evidence-based practice has become synonymous with robustness and quality.

The value of quantitative evidence is that it provides good indicators of the outcomes of various treatment options which can be compared against one another to determine the most effective intervention. The value of qualitative evidence is that it provides a mechanism for investigating the processes whereby these outcomes are achieved.

A   **Activity   Reflecting on your views**

Different professionals have their own perspectives on evidence-based practice and whether this should be quantitative or qualitative. If you are going to undertake a qualitative project in child mental health it is important that you take time to reflect on your personal beliefs about the value of evidence in your discipline.

The need for evidence in child mental health

In mental health the value of evidence has been hierarchically organised in terms of the perceived usefulness to inform practice (Rishel, 2007). This has meant that quantitative evidence has dominated our understanding of mental health. Indeed this can be helpful and can provide an overview of statistical prevalence of child mental health difficulties. It can also demonstrate the comparative effectiveness of one form of treatment over another. This is often referred to as 'outcomes research'.

Although quantitative researchers use methods such as observations, experiments and questionnaires, in health the most desired method is the randomised controlled trial (RCT). Unfortunately this hierarchy of evidence tends to favour quantitative evidence, often neglecting the value of qualitative work (Davies et al., 2000). This highlights a problem with the dominance of evidence produced by RCTs. This is not to say that RCTs are inherently bad, they are extremely important for generating evidence, but it is helpful to recognise that other methods produce different types of evidence that are also necessary for the advancement of knowledge.

Evidence on effective treatments, outcomes and prevention in mental health is necessary for funding and commissioning of services. However, research needs to transcend outcomes, as attention to process in child mental health is also essential (Rishel, 2007) and qualitative research is often referred to as 'process research'. In its simplest form, qualitative evidence can help us to understand the children's experiences and provide us with insight into their needs, feelings and perceptions. By utilising qualitative methods professionals can learn what it feels like to experience a mental health difficulty. They can use this insight to better appreciate the nature of the individual's experience and enable them to treat and communicate with that person in a more sensitive way (Kearney, 2001).

As you become familiar with the literature you will notice that there is little data available about children's expectations/experiences of mental health difficulties or services. Qualitative approaches to research can help to address this gap as they afford the opportunity for a high degree of discovery and the possibility of generating new theories (Kearney, 2001). Practitioners are now starting to be more critical of the research evidence they engage with and are better skilled to question whether all aspects of health and illness can be readily quantified (Thorne, 2009). The use of qualitative approaches therefore, is becoming much more accepted. Consider the difference between the two cases below.

Case example: Value of evidence Case 1

Ciaran is a consultant child psychiatrist working in a mental health service. He has been commissioned as part of a team to test whether a manualised treatment for anxiety is better than the standard treatment.

A   Activity   Choosing a form of evidence

Which type of evidence is Ciaran trying to produce? Is the RCT appropriate here?

Case example: Value of evidence Case 2

Sabine is a speech and language therapist who has an interest in autism. She wants to explore how older children describe their problems and whether parents have a different perspective.

A   Activity   Choosing a form of evidence

What type of evidence is Sabine trying to produce? Is the RCT appropriate here?

It should seem clear that Ciaran's project is well suited to a RCT as Ciaran is trying to establish the effectiveness of an intervention. Sabine, however, is more interested in the experiences of families to discover differences in how parents and children make sense of the symptoms. In choosing the design for her project, Sabine could conduct either a quantitative or qualitative approach. However, as a speech and language therapist Sabine is interested in the specific communication practices engaged in by parents and children during clinical interventions and is therefore much more likely to choose a qualitative method.

 Remember that your own research project may contribute to the evidence-base. It is important to be clear about which approach is appropriate to meet your aims.

Performing a literature search

An important element of understanding evidence is searching the literature. A literature review is a systematic method for identifying, evaluating and synthesising evidence (Fink, 2005). During planning you will need to narrow down the focus of your project. When you first start exploring the literature you may feel a little overwhelmed by the volume of evidence on any particular mental health condition or area. However, by searching the literature effectively you will be able to expose any gaps in the knowledge (Robson, 2011).

 Your literature search should include all elements of your project and this means that you need to read about methods, as well as about your topic (Blaxter et al., 2001).

Table 2.1 provides a useful practical strategy for performing a literature search.

A good way to start is to write down your key words and present them in groups of three. Put these into Google Scholar for a general search and then into more focused electronic databases for a specialised search. There are many databases that exist and you can access these online. Good ones for mental health are EBSCO, SAGE, SCOPUS, MEDline, PsychINFO and ERIC. The key words are essential for determining the success of your search. See the case example below.

Table 2.1   Practical hints for performing literature searches

	Practical hint
First	Make sure your project is tightly defined to help you judge which areas of the literature are most relevant.
Second	Speak to your team, colleagues, supervisor or other experts in the field to get advice. These people will often provide you with a good article to start with, and you can use the reference list in this to help you identify other relevant sources.
Third	A useful place to start your general search is the web-engine Google Scholar. This allows you to type in whole sentences and searches the relevant academic literature.
Fourth	Consult electronic databases. These typically involve either the input of key words to search or you can search by subject. They are more refined searches and more discipline specific.
Fifth	Remember that journal articles are not the only source of evidence. It is important to consider books, newspaper articles, credible web sources and confessional accounts.
Sixth	When reading from books it is useful to photocopy the chapter so that you can make notes in the margins and use highlighter pens (please abide by the photocopying legislation, though!).

Case example: Key words

Katie has taken a new post as a community psychiatric nurse. Her role requires her to do research. She is interested in how children diagnosed with a mental health difficulty feel about taking their medication when they are going through changes associated with adolescence. She plans to conduct semi-structured interviews. Her research question is 'How do older children with mental health difficulties and their parents perceive the effectiveness of medication?'

Katie needs to be sure that there is not already lots of evidence in this area. She also feels that her question needs refining so she undertakes a literature search.

Using Google Scholar Katie typed the words 'mental health' and 'medication'.

 Activity   Katie's search terms

What is your opinion of Katie's search terms? Do you think that Katie managed to get the articles she needed for her research? Try typing in these two terms into Google Scholar yourself.

A broad search of the literature can be useful early on as it allows researchers to learn more about the topic before deciding which elements are most useful for their research (Creswell, 2003). If you are still unsure how to narrow down your own ideas, then doing a broad literature search might help you identify specific issues that are underrepresented.

Case example: Key words (part 2)

When Katie performed her Google Scholar search it returned 872,000 results! This told Katie two things:

1. Her project was too broadly focused.
2. Her key search terms were too broad.

In consultation with her supervisor Katie decided to be more focused and more defined in her search. Following an interesting article in her local newspaper about ADHD Katie decided to narrow her research to this particular disorder and generated the new question of 'How do older children with ADHD and their parents perceive the value and effectiveness of medication?'

She entered the search terms 'ADHD' and 'Medication' into Google Scholar and it still returned 73,900 results on that day. Clearly Katie needed to narrow down her choice of key terms for her search, but also needed to think about the relevance of these results.

 Activity   Katie's search terms (part 2)

What terms do you think Katie should use to help her narrow down her search?

There are lots of different combinations of words that Katie can use to search the literature for relevant evidence. For example she could combine lots of different sequences of terms, such as:

- Adolescents, medication, ADHD
- Medication, ADHD, qualitative
- Effectiveness, medication, ADHD

 Because of the multitude of terms you might want to include in your search it is important you write down what you have searched for to avoid repetition.

Conversely some students may find that when they enter their search terms there are no *relevant* articles returned. This may reflect that there has been little previous research, but more likely it will mean that you need to broaden your search. Find general articles in the field/area that interests you, but that perhaps have used different methods. Remember in the unlikely event you find the exact study you are planning it may mean your work is not original so you may need to change it. An alternative way of searching for articles within the electronic databases is to use the built-in thesaurus. The thesaurus is a controlled vocabulary which provides a consistent way to retrieve information across fields that may use different terms for the same concept (Fink, 2005).

Example

In the electronic database PsychINFO the thesaurus is used and in MEDLINE it is defined by the Medical Subjects Headings (MeSH).

This brings up a list of words you can search by. You can 'check' multiple terms from this list for the database to search. Other databases are similar to this.

As you progress through your literature search you should assess whether to read the articles you find. To do this you will need to read the abstracts. You may find that you read lots of abstracts but only actually save/print a small number of articles. The abstract, if it is well written, should tell you what the topic is, what the researchers did, found and concluded and what the broader implications of their findings are.

 It is highly unlikely that you will be able to read all of the results returned from your search and therefore you need to consider which articles are worth reading.

Once you have your collection you need to read them and make critical notes. Reading is an important and informative exercise but it is better if you engage in critical reading and critical note-taking (Blaxter et al., 2001).

How to read a journal article

To critically read a qualitative paper you need to be questioning whether the paper is describing an important problem, whether the methodology is appropriate to address that problem and whether the researcher's perspective is included (Greenhalgh & Taylor, 1997). Part of the difficulty for readers of qualitative work is that the term 'qualitative' is an umbrella term for a heterogeneous group of methodologies and different types of research questions need to be appraised in different ways (Kuper et al., 2008).

It is necessary to read these articles in a critical way, which is a two-phase process:

1.   Read the article.
2.   Read the article again but make critical notes.

This may feel time-consuming but it is a good strategy for ensuring you fully engage with it.

 Remember that critical reading is not just about finding fault but also about assessing the strength of the argument and the evidence presented.

When you are reading through a child mental health article remember that many mental health issues are associated with different and sometimes contentious points of view, so it is important that you acknowledge any biases and attempt to present balanced perspectives.

Example

Consider this article on complementary interventions, which for autism can be controversial. The article reports some negative views and the authors needed to present a balanced discourse whilst maintaining the professionals' perspectives.

O'Reilly, M., Cook, L. & Karim, K. (2012). Complementary or controversial care? The opinions of professionals on complementary and alternative interventions for Autistic Spectrum Disorder. *Clinical Child Psychology and Psychiatry*, e-pub = doi: 10.1177/1359104511435340.

 Activity   Neutrality

We recommend you read this article to explore how the authors managed the balanced view.

Making critical notes

When you start writing critically you should provide a clear assessment of the argument presented and recognise any limitations of it. To do this effectively you will need to weigh up the strength of that argument compared with those put forward by others. Each paper should inform you about what type of study was conducted and you will need to make some critical decisions regarding whether the design was appropriate (Greenhalgh, 1997). There are a number of steps for developing critical notes. We outline the preliminary steps in Table 2.2, the main steps in Table 2.3 and final steps in Table 2.4.

Table 2.2   Initial steps for critiquing a paper

	Critical steps
Step 1	Write down the full reference for the paper. This may seem obvious but it is easy to lose the reference later. You may prefer to use computer software such as RefWorks to help you do this.
Step 2	Read the abstract and note the key points from it. It can be useful to copy and paste the full abstract from the database into your notes as well as writing key bullet points.
Step 3	Contextualise the paper by reading through the introduction section. This will help you see what literature the author felt was relevant and will give you a sense of the argument. This can also help you to identify additional papers that you might want to read. Note down key points made and try to write a summary of the argument presented.

Table 2.3   Main steps for critiquing a paper

	Critical steps
Step 4	Identify the aims of the study and write these down. You will need this for later when determining whether the authors met their aims and objectives. The article should aim to make some contribution to the field of child mental health and you should be clear what this is.
Step 5	Read through the methodology section and identify any limitations with it. Write these down in a list. Consider whether the setting for the data collection was justified, and whether there is a clear rationale for the data collection method.
Step 6	Look at the recruitment strategy and consider whether it is appropriate to meet the aims. Consider how the children were selected and whether that was appropriate for the design.
Step 7	Read the section on ethics. Consider how well ethics have been addressed and remember that child mental health research invokes particular ethical sensitivities which should be considered.
Step 8	Read through the results/analysis/findings section. Think about how well they are reported, whether they are understandable, whether the narrative/statistics are clear, whether they relate to the research question/hypothesis asked. You might want to summarise the key findings for your notes.

Table 2.4 Final steps for critiquing a paper

	Critical steps
Step 9	Identify the author's main conclusions and see if they tie up with the aims and objectives identified earlier. Consider whether we now know something important about this particular child mental health difficulty or area.
Step 10	Summarise the critique and identify the core strengths of the argument and the key limitations of it. Think about whether this research article is useful to you in your practice or research with children.

The general critical appraisal part of your notes is particularly important as this will help inform anything you write later and will demonstrate your understanding of the paper as a whole.

 Remember you need to ensure any literature you read is either historically important or up-to-date.

Arguments for quality

To develop your ability to be critical of research it is helpful to have some appreciation of the different quality frameworks against which research is judged. The arguments about quality in quantitative research are more straightforward than for qualitative, as quantitative research tends to be judged against three fundamental markers:

- *Validity* – refers to the extent to which the study sets out to measure what it intended to measure.
- *Reliability* – refers to the extent to which the study can be replicated by others.
- *Generalisability* – refers to the extent to which the findings are applicable to populations beyond the participants.

In quantitative research it is important that your research has validity and reliability and that you are able to generalise your results to the broader population. This means that your research should measure what it sets out to measure (validity). Note however, that although we do not go into detail here, there are many different types of validity. It is also important that your study is reliable, that is, it could be carried out again by a different researcher. It should produce similar results under different conditions. Finally, you should be able to generalise your results. This means that your results should apply beyond the conditions under which you conducted your research to a wider population.

Part of the problem for producing quality criteria for qualitative work relates to a debate about whether to use the same quality criteria that is used to judge quantitative research (Mays & Pope, 2000). This has led to two distinct positions:

Position 1: There are researchers who argue that qualitative research represents a distinct paradigm from quantitative research and different quality criteria are needed to assess it.

Position 2: There are researchers who argue that the difference in philosophy between qualitative and quantitative research is not sufficient to require distinctive quality assessment criteria.

Some researchers who argue that quality criteria are needed for qualitative research have adapted the quantitative notions of quality to fit with the qualitative paradigm. These researchers have argued that we can adapt the three core notions of quality and apply them to qualitative research differently:

- Validity in qualitative research relates to the transparency of the claims made by the researcher (Perakyla, 2004). This means that validity relates to the credibility and trustworthiness of the claims made. In other words it is important that researchers in the reporting of their qualitative research are transparent about the process and the interpretations made.
- Reliability in qualitative work is also more complex. Reliability relates to the extent to which replication of the study is possible. However, because of the differences in different qualitative approaches, this kind of reliability can be difficult to achieve. Reliability in qualitative work is therefore referred to more often as consistency and relates to whether all qualitative researchers would discover the same kinds of issues as others if given similar participants in similar circumstances (LeCompte & Goetz, 1982).
- Overall, therefore, the quality of qualitative work is determined by its credibility. To achieve credibility the study must have transferability (the extent to which findings can be transferred to other settings), dependability (the extent to which further research would produce similar findings if carried out as described in the study) and confirmability (evidence of the claims made) (Lincoln & Guba, 1985).

Other researchers argue that qualitative research methods are distinctive and that simply applying and adapting the general quality markers of quantitative approaches is inappropriate. Despite many agreeing that distinctive criteria are needed, if you look at the literature, you will notice that there is little consensus regarding how to judge quality in qualitative work. This is because of two further differences of opinion within the research community:

Position 1: There are those who argue that we need a universal check-list for quality for all qualitative approaches.

Position 2: There are those who argue that because of the heterogeneity within this paradigm, universal criteria are implausible.

Evidently the epistemological scope of qualitative work is simply too broad for a single set of criteria to be developed (Sandleowski & Barroso, 2002). There has, however, been increasing pressure to formalise quality standards, produce frameworks and provide guidance for qualitative researchers (Spencer et al., 2003). This has been in response to funding requirements and ethical review. This is particularly pertinent in health research as the complexity of the debate makes it difficult for practitioners to evaluate the usefulness of existing studies (Devers, 1999). There has therefore been an uneasy compromise in the literature with the development of several guiding frameworks for judging quality. Many of these express some caution regarding their universality, noting that each different qualitative methodology still needs to be judged against its own specific quality markers.

Summary

In this chapter we have contextualised the need for research in child mental health and illustrated the importance of translating this evidence into practice. By differentiating outcomes from processes we have explicated the ways in which qualitative research can provide the depth of knowledge about the processes of clinical interventions that make them effective. The value of the qualitative evidence-base therefore is in its ability to demonstrate how and why particular interventions are effective and not simply illuminating what works. Thus the value of the evidence-base rests on its quality, although judging the quality of qualitative work is best considered in relation to the particular methodology chosen.

Key messages

- Child mental health research is necessary due to the rise in child mental health needs and the greater demand on services.
- Qualitative research can be beneficial in demonstrating the processes involved in effective child mental health interventions.
- A literature review requires a systematic approach.
- Judging quality in qualitative research is best managed by alignment with the quality criteria for that particular methodology.

Further reading

Hoagwood, K., Burns, B., Kiser, L., Ringeisem, H. & Schoenwald, S. (2001). Evidence-based practice in child and adolescent mental health services. *Psychiatric Services, 52*(9), 1179–1189.

Kearney, M. (2001). Levels and applications of qualitative research evidence. *Research in Nursing and Health, 24*, 145–153.

Waddell, C. & Godderis, R. (2005). Rethinking evidence-based practice for children's mental health. *Evidence Based Mental Health, 8*, 60–62.

CHAPTER 3

CLINICAL AND RESEARCH ROLES

Learning outcomes

- Recognise the impact that your multiple roles may have on the research process.
- Recognise the tension between the clinical and researcher role.
- Appreciate how your role may influence the asymmetry between you and your child participants.
- Identify the ways in which roles can lead to coercion and/or exploitation in the research context.

Introduction

We open this chapter by discussing the different roles you may occupy when doing research with children who have mental health difficulties. You will inhabit a number of roles in your life, such as 'clinician', 'teacher', 'social worker', 'trainee', 'parent', 'researcher', and these can impact on the way you conduct your research. Problems may arise when a tension occurs between two or more of your roles and in research in mental health this is most likely to be between your professional role as a clinical, educational, social work practitioner or trainee and that of researcher. In this chapter we highlight when and where this tension may occur and provide practical strategies for managing the ways in which this may influence the research relationship.

In this chapter we also deal with issues of power, professional skills and potential conflicts of interest. We consider how different professional titles may elicit different responses from children and how this may affect your findings. We explore how researching one's own clients/pupils may involve different dynamics and provide advice about how to work reflectively to avoid asymmetry becoming coercive.

The impact of role on research

The research relationship you build with your participants is important (Freeman & Mathison, 2009) as is the way you present yourself to them. Your profession and role will impact the way children see you and may influence their expectations about you in terms of what expertise you have and how you might interact with them.

A   Activity   Your roles

Write down all the roles you occupy as this may be useful later. Include any personal as well as professional roles that might influence the way you conduct your research.

It is important to think about how you introduce yourself to parents and children. Research indicates that the way you introduce yourself is significant, as is the title you use.

Example

If you introduce yourself as a doctor, it is likely that participants (or parents) will ask you clinical questions, or apologise for any negative views of the service. If you introduce yourself as a researcher, the participants are likely to be more open to you and more talkable about their perceptions of services (see Richards & Emslie, 2000).

Of course there are different types of doctors and many health professionals do not carry this title. However, you will probably have a professional role that you usually use to introduce yourself by. If you are a qualified psychotherapist, teacher, nurse or social worker for example, introducing yourself in this way may result in questions linked to your profession. It is therefore important that you give serious consideration to both how you introduce yourself in person and in your documents (such as participant information sheets and consent forms).

 Be careful to give full and appropriate information to your participants. If you represent more than one institution it may be necessary to point this out.

Dual roles

When conducting research with children about mental health then there are two roles that are most relevant, practitioner and researcher. Four issues linked to dual role are outlined in Table 3.1.

Engaging children/families as participants is different and your role/title has potential to influence the process in many ways. There are some similarities particularly between clinical practice and qualitative data collection which can blur some of the boundaries. Both therapeutic and research relationships require a telling of experiences whereby one individual reports and the other listens, with the listener attempting to make sense of, interpret,

Table 3.1   Four issues of dual role

Conducting research with these participants	Description
Your own clients/pupils	It is common for professionals/trainees to undertake research which involves their own clients/pupils and this raises particular issues in relation to dual role.
Children who are in your service/institution	Even if you choose to exclude children whom you see yourself, it is possible you may conduct research with children who are seen by your colleagues and this can still raise issues in relation to dual role.
Children outside of your service/institution	Although the impact may be softened by recruiting children from a service/institution that you do not work for, your role, title and expertise can still impact on your participants' perception of you and therefore the data you collect.
Other professionals or your peers	Not all child mental health research will involve children directly and you may choose to interview other professionals in your field. It is likely that practitioners from the same or different professional backgrounds will respond to you differently.

reframe and understand those stories (Hart & Crawford-Wright, 1999). It is important to bear in mind that the goals and objectives of clinical practice are different from the goals and objectives of research and sometimes these conflict. In clinical practice the professional is charged with pursuing the client's best interests whereas in research the researcher focuses on issues of scientific acceptability and research integrity (Hart & Crawford-Wright, 1999).

Valuable knowledge can also be gained through collecting data from staff working in child mental health and if you choose to employ them as your participant group then you must be careful how you present yourself and your role to them. Research indicates that some professionals feel they may be judged by the researcher or that the data collection is a test of their knowledge (Coar & Sim, 2006).

In practice child mental health practitioners promote the welfare of children, but researchers have a priority to meet the aims of the research. In Table 3.2, we illustrate this possible conflict of interests and some of the main difficulties of occupying dual roles in research.

Although it is difficult to eliminate these problems entirely, with careful planning it is possible to reduce the likelihood or impact of them:

- *Therapeutic and research boundaries*: Set boundaries in the research relationship and afford some distance from the participants. Make the boundaries clear at the beginning of the data collection process (Dickson-Swift et al., 2006).
- *Incompatibility of expectations*: Make it clear that you will not be giving participants medical/therapeutic/social/educational advice and illustrate in simple, child-friendly terms what your role is in the research and the purpose of it.

Table 3.2 Potential problems in the dual relationship

Problem	Description
Boundary drift	Qualitative research techniques can have some therapeutic benefit for participants and researchers may find maintaining the boundaries difficult (Dickson-Swift et al., 2006). Encouraging participants to talk openly risks turning data collection into a therapeutic session.
Incompatibility of expectations	The participants may frame their expectations of you on the basis of the professional role you occupy and this may increase the potential for misunderstanding where expectations are not carefully managed (Kitchener, 1988).
Possible distress	Clinically trained researchers have the skills to negotiate sensitive topics, which makes their data more person-centred. However this risks over-disclosure and distress as participants are invited to tell their stories (Hart & Crawford-Wright, 1999).
Trust and coercion	Ostensibly a trusting relationship has potential to encourage recruitment to research. By engaging one's own clients in research there is already a relationship in place which can foster more open research data collection. Your role therefore may invoke trust in the children but risks coercing them into participating (Etherington, 1996).

- *Expertise and authority*: Children inevitably will see you as an adult with authority and potentially with expertise. It is useful to soften this power difference by allowing children some control over the research process.
- *Emotional distress*: If you have clinical expertise then you may have skills to elicit more information from participants than non-clinical researchers. It is essential that you are self-aware and do not overly encourage children to disclose more than they may be comfortable with, or can be managed in the setting.
- *Trust*: With self-awareness you can largely avoid abuse of the trust your participants have in you. However, it may still be wise to ask a different member of the team to take consent rather than asking children yourself.

If you are occupying a dual role and have to take consent and collect the data yourself then the issue of trust is important as there may be a real conflict of interests. You should pay attention to the potential influence that you may have over children in the research context on the basis of your professional title, or existing relationship with them.

 These subtle hierarchies, foundation of trust and expectations of authority and expertise have potential for exploitation and coercion of participants.

Professional case example: Interview with Dr Muskett

Dr Tom Muskett has written extensively on child mental health, particularly on autism. We asked him some questions about the challenges of being a speech and language therapist while undertaking research.

1 In what ways does your role as a speech and language therapist facilitate your research in child mental health?

My roles in practice and clinical education are invaluable for my research, fundamentally because they enable continuous in-action reflection on the implications of my research for practice, and indeed the implications of practice for my research. My research tends to be critical, qualitative and relatively small scale, and therefore may not immediately be recognised as 'clinically relevant' in the current healthcare culture. However, being able to understand reflexively how it links to facets of contemporary practice enables me to identify who my work might be of interest to, and how best to communicate it.

2 How do you manage the sometimes competing roles of researcher and clinician?

This can be difficult in my case, because some of the research I am interested in can challenge taken-for-granted ways of thinking about mental health and mental health diagnoses. To manage this conflict, I have always tried to remain engaged with a variety of different research approaches and traditions across health and social sciences. This cross-disciplinary grounding enables me to understand clinical practice from several different perspectives at the same time, which has helped reduce any competition between these roles.

3 What would you advise clinicians who are new to research regarding the issue of dual role?

My advice would be to ensure that you have a broad and solid understanding of the methods and approaches that underpin 'mainstream' research in child mental health, regardless of whether you wish to conduct this kind of research or not. This allows you to understand key political and practice drivers and research themes, and – crucially – how your own work might relate to these. Even if you do not want to do 'mainstream' research, you will find it highly beneficial to be able to describe what you do want to do in such terms.

Some useful references

Muskett, T., Body, R. & Perkins, M. (2012). Uncovering the dynamic in static assessment interaction. *Child Language Teaching Therapy, 28,* 87–99.
Muskett, T., Perkins, P., Clegg, J. & Body, R. (2010). Inflexibility as an interactional phenomenon: Using conversation analysis to re-examine a symptom of autism. *Clinical Linguistics and Phonetics, 24,* 1–16.
There is more on his website: www.shef.ac.uk/hcs/staff/muskett

Asymmetry and roles

We have illustrated that a concern when conducting research with children who have mental health difficulties is their understanding of the relationships which exist between you and them. When conducting this type of research there are ethical considerations to be aware of which arise mostly from the inherent power imbalance between professional/client (pupil) and researcher/ participant. The most prominent issue in relation to dual roles is that this duality creates a power differential on several levels as described in Table 3.3.

Table 3.3 Power relationships

Relationship	Description
Adult/child	Although there are historical and cultural influences affecting the way childhood is conceptualised, in most contemporary societies it is accepted that there is an inherent power difference between adults and children.
Researcher/participant	It is generally understood that there is an asymmetry between researchers and their participants.
Mental health practitioner/ client (patient)	When occupying a dual role this may be the most challenging asymmetry to minimise. There is power imbalance between the 'expert' professional role and the client or patient being treated.
Health advantage/ health disadvantage	Individuals with mental health difficulties are typically understood to be in a less powerful position by nature of the fact that they are experiencing impairment in their functioning and are therefore less able.

As explained, your dual role has potential to increase risks of exploitation (Kitchener, 1988) and understanding these dynamics will help you to be more reflective in your research.

First, recognise that your status as an adult may impact on the research process with children. Traditionally in society there is an unequal societal power relationship between adults and children (Holt, 2004). Children spend much of their time in various personal/institutional contexts being told what to do and how to behave by adults. It is likely that children will either want to please you or be wary of you, as you are another adult entering their social world. It is necessary that you engage in children's culture as a way of representing their views as accurately as possible and be self-aware of the hierarchical difference that the adult/child status creates (Holt, 2004).

 Listening to children can be time-consuming, but you still need to respect and listen to their views (Clark, 2005).

Second, you need to understand that your role as researcher and the child's role as participant create asymmetry. The researcher's 'power' lies in the fact that they determine the aims, methods, types of data collected and the knowledge produced (Gallagher, 2008). By virtue of your role as a researcher it is you who gets to make most of the decisions (Etherington, 2001). Those who are being studied may, by virtue of their race, class, age, ability or socio-economic status, be potentially marginalised to some extent by their exclusion from the process of knowledge production (Gallagher, 2008). It is arguable that you have a responsibility to your participants to empower them during this process (Etherington, 2001).

Children do have some power in the research process as they have the power to give/decline consent/assent and the power to withdraw. It is up to you to ensure they can exercise it.

Third, be aware of the asymmetry created by virtue of your role as a professional, which is especially pertinent in child mental health research. Because of the trust that is created by your role/title (particularly with your own clients/pupils), there is potential for exploitation. The power your role affords means that you may inadvertently coerce children into agreeing to participate in your research. If you are inexperienced or have vested interest in your project you may be unaware of your influence. It is important therefore that you take a reflective position on this and constantly check your motives, communication style and research techniques. It may also be useful to consult with your colleagues and supervisor regarding the strategies you are using.

 Do not forget to consider this during the data collection as well as at the consent stage.

Fourth, there is asymmetry between those who are mentally healthy and those who are not. The concepts of mental health difficulties and mental illness are associated with notions of discrimination, stigma and powerlessness and this is not limited to those with a diagnosis or accessing services (Kidd & Finlayson, 2006). It is important that you consider this in your research and ensure that you are not contributing to stigma or negative views. Young people typically view mental ill health negatively and have to manage the dilemma of being associated with mental health difficulties (O'Reilly, Taylor et al., 2009). You therefore need to pay attention to the terms you are using in the research process and work on ways of enabling these children's voices to be heard and listened to.

 Parents often feel uninformed regarding the cause, diagnosis and outcome of their child's condition (Garth & Aroni, 2003) and may use the research process as an opportunity to seek answers from you.

Remember that power is typically seen as a commodity possessed by dominant groups but bear in mind that this view tends to obscure the complex multi-layered nature of power in terms of how it is exercised within the research space (Gallagher, 2008).

Example

Maya is undertaking a master's degree in forensic psychology and is in the process of doing her dissertation. She is interested in obtaining the opinions of teenage boys on whether drug and alcohol abuse impacts on mental health and crime. She brings together small groups to discuss this. To empower them she makes sure that she allows the boys to lead the discussion, provides activities such as photographs to stimulate discussion and makes it clear she is not a figure of authority. During the data collection she encounters a problem and comes to you, as her supervisor, to discuss it. During her first focus group a fight broke out between two boys as Pablo accused Eduardo of lying about his cannabis usage. Hostility between the two boys was commonly known amongst the children but not to Maya. As the fight escalated and became physical, Maya struggled to regain control of the group and a passing teacher stepped in.

A   **Activity   Helping Maya**

What issues of asymmetry may be operating here and what could Maya do?

It is clear from this case study that there does need to be a balance between the power of the researcher and that of the children. There are different issues of asymmetry operating here:

1. Gender – it is often the case that there can be a power difference between men and women. Maya is a female doing research with males, even though they are younger than she is.
2. Researcher/participant – as a researcher Maya has a powerful position, but she worked hard to diminish this.
3. Adult/child – these are older children growing into adults and therefore have more power than younger children, but as an adult Maya still has an adult authority.
4. Health – the children selected for this research did not specifically have mental health difficulties, rather this was the focus of the conversation.

Maya clearly struggled to take charge of the situation as it unfolded and in her enthusiasm to reduce the power differentials between her and the boys she perhaps afforded them too much power. Striking a balance is a delicate endeavour and Maya could have set out a 'contract' at the beginning of the group to stipulate acceptable and unacceptable behaviour. It would also have been useful if Maya had communicated better in the planning stages so as to avoid bringing together boys who had a history of conflict with one another and also ensured that there was a teacher or other responsible adult at hand to take the authoritarian/disciplinarian role so that Maya could be free to not have to take on this role as well.

Summary

In this chapter we have discussed some issues pertinent to the multiple roles you may occupy. The nature of your role/title has potential to impact on the ethical sensitivities of the project, the consent process and data collection. We have therefore provided you with some practical guidance related to how to manage this. In the chapter we have illustrated that there may be a conflict of interest or tension between your professional role and your role as a researcher. This shows that it is necessary to appreciate how your roles can influence the asymmetry between you and your child participants and how this raises issues related to coercion and power.

Key messages

- If you are engaged in child mental health research then it is likely that you will have several roles, including adult, clinician/teacher/social worker and researcher.
- Sometimes there is a tension between these different roles.
- Your professional skills have potential to unduly influence children in terms of coercing them to participate and encouraging disclosure which they may not be comfortable with.
- It is important to recognise the power differences that the different roles create.

Further reading

Christensen, P. (2004). Children's participation in ethnographic research: issues of power and representation, *Children and Society*, *18*, 165–176.

Kitchener, K. (1988). Dual role relationships – what makes them so problematic? *Journal of Counseling and Development*, *67*, 217–221.

Richards, H. & Emslie, C. (2000). The 'doctor' or the 'girl from the University'? Considering the influence of professional roles on qualitative interviewing. *Family Practice*, *17*(10), 71–75.

CHAPTER 4

ETHICS IN CHILD MENTAL HEALTH RESEARCH

Learning outcomes

- Appreciate why ethics are important in child mental health research.
- Distinguish between the ethical paradigms.
- Appreciate the process of ethical regulation.
- Identify the four core principles of ethics.
- Differentiate how these apply to these principles to qualitative work with children.

Introduction

In this chapter we consider issues pertinent to research ethics in child mental health. There are different approaches to ethics in research which are underpinned by philosophical ideas and to help you understand these we differentiate the broad ideologies. The chapter contextualises these ideas by considering the important process of ethical regulation and review. We provide you with some practical guiding principles to communicate with ethics committees and consider some of the ways in which you might approach ethical regulation. The latter part of this chapter focuses on the practical application of ethics by considering the main four ethical principles. Here we guide you through some of the complexities of acting in an ethically appropriate way by considering some of the principles of informed consent, the importance of equality, boundaries of confidentiality, challenges of child protection and some of the specific ethical sensitivities that doing qualitative research invokes.

Why ethics are important

The purpose of child research is to gather information that aims to improve the lives of children with mental health difficulties and/or their families. This means that researchers should be working within a framework that ensures that there is no harm caused to those participating in research. An overarching consideration in research then is to maintain a stance which enables you to take a reflective position on weighing up the benefits and risks associated with your project. This is essential when doing research with children who have mental health difficulties, particularly as child mental health research is relatively new in comparison to adult mental health (Hoagwood et al., 1996).

 Activity   Why are ethics important?

Before you read further try to write down three reasons why you think it is important to act in an ethical way in research with children with mental health difficulties.

Benefits and risks

Whilst the aim of research is to benefit participants and/or society, there are inherent risks in any form of research (Barke, 2009). In order to capitalise on the benefits the potential risks need to be weighed up. Although research does not always have direct benefit to those who participate (Wilson & Hunter, 2010), a poorly designed study has limited possibility of any benefit (Fisher et al., 2002). If you take an ethical approach to your research it will help you safeguard against detrimental impact on your participants.

Protecting children

Ethics are important to protect participants from harm. Ultimately it is your responsibility to ensure the safety of your participants (Field & Behrman, 2004). Although this is important in quantitative research, particularly where they may be exposed to physical risks, in qualitative research there are different potential risks that should be considered. In general terms this relates to issues regarding confidentiality and protecting participants' identity. The open style of qualitative work creates an environment whereby rich and interesting data can be collected but at the same time increases the possibility of levels of disclosure that quantitative research is less likely to generate.

Reducing risks of exploitation

Children are often viewed as vulnerable and in need of protection from researchers who may exploit them (Morrow & Richards, 1996). Be careful to consider how involved the child is in the research process so as to mitigate the possibility of coercion or exploitation. One way to avoid this is to foster a collaborative relationship with child participants to enable them to be involved in shaping the research agenda (Thomas & O'Kane, 1998). Additionally those with mental health difficulties are positioned as vulnerable and researchers should be aware of this ensuring careful safety monitoring, consultation with relevant gatekeepers and enhanced informed consent procedures (DuBois, 2008).

Reputation, trust and credibility

It is important to be ethical because your own reputation as a credible researcher will rest upon your professionalism. Your personal conduct as a researcher will also reflect on the institution that you represent and the wider research community. It is important to remember that participants put their trust in institutions with the belief that they have regulations designed to protect their safety (Melo-Martin & Ho, 2008). Therefore being trusted to work within an ethically sound framework has potential to promote the value of research more publicly. This is especially important as mental health research may involve sensitive or potentially stigmatising questions (DuBois, 2008).

Taking power and responsibility seriously

An important issue for researchers relates to the disparity in status and power between adults and children (Morrow & Richards, 1996). As an ethical researcher you need to work to redress the unequal power balance by ensuring that all individuals share in the process by being respected and listened to (Flewitt, 2005). An ethical approach to knowledge generation by conducting research is to place more emphasis on children as active social agents and not simply passive subjects (Woodhead & Faulkner, 2000).

Ensuring the researcher has considered his/her impact on participants

This issue is more pertinent in qualitative research as the focus of qualitative research is to elicit information from the participant. You need to be mindful that you are integral to the process of collecting that data and therefore it is important that you reflect on the personal impact you may have on the participant. You need to bear in mind that children's responses are provided within a context and in response to questions by an individual. Therefore individual characteristics of the researcher such as status, age, gender and ethnicity may be relevant for consideration.

The process of ethical regulation

Risk and uncertainty in research has led to the development of governance frameworks established to ensure compliance with ethical, legal, professional and scientific standards (Kerrison et al., 2003). Ethical review is now mandatory for research in many countries (Dixon-Woods et al., 2007) and the role of the committee is to protect both research participants and the researcher (Morrow & Richards, 1996). Its central purpose is to agree a decision regarding the ethical feasibility of a proposed project and this will be conveyed in writing (O'Reilly, Dixon-Woods et al., 2009).

While there are differences in the format and process of ethics regulation across countries, there are some elements of the procedure for obtaining approval for research which are generally universal. We outline these in Figure 4.1.

Although the advent of research governance has been of benefit in assuring adherence to ethical principles in research, responsibility for managing research risk and protecting children is shared by ethical review bodies and researchers (Carter, 2009). Any research which involves recruiting participants from vulnerable groups and/or addressing sensitive topics will be treated more cautiously by ethics committees. This is because ethics committees work on the premise that certain categories of people may be more likely to be exploited and require special protection (Levine et al., 2004).

However, qualitative research evolves as the project unfolds and this is often difficult to predict, which can make it more challenging to make specific

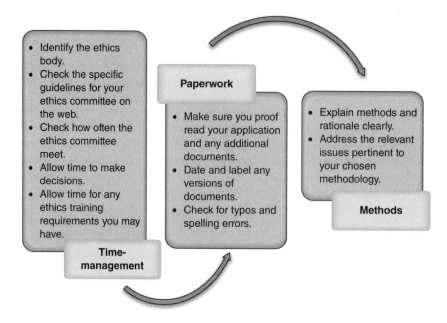

Figure 4.1   Process of ethics

enough predictions to satisfy ethics committee criteria. Many qualitative projects are granted approval, however, and if changes are necessary then these can be revisited with the committee (Alderson, 2007). Usually if any major amendments are made during your project then these will need to be resubmitted to the original ethics committee for review. Researchers have a particular responsibility to ensure that the ethical principles are applied throughout all stages of the research process (Flewitt, 2005).

Ethical approaches

The process of ethics in child mental health is iterative. This means that ethical considerations do not end once you have gained ethical approval from a committee, but are revisited continuously throughout the process.

 Activity   Reflections on ethics

Before you go any further it may be useful to think about your own position regarding what you think are the important issues to consider in undertaking an ethically viable project.

There are three broad moral philosophies which inform the ethical approaches adopted in research and these are usefully discussed in Beauchamp and Childress (2008). These are consequentialism, deontology and virtue ethics. We present a brief overview of these in Table 4.1, but focus on deontology as this is the most commonly used in health research.

Table 4.1   Approaches to ethics

Approach	Description
Consequentialism	Less concerned with the motivations of the researcher. Focuses on the consequences of actions.
Deontology	A rules-based (principles) approach. Less concerned with consequences and more concerned with the nature of actions.
Virtue ethics	More concerned with the moral characteristics of the researcher.

Most often in health and social sciences an adherence to the deontological approach as a mechanism for making every effort to avoid harm to participants is taken. The four principles of deontology are to respect autonomy, endorse beneficence, ensure non-maleficence and promote justice, and we deal with each of these in turn.

The four principles

The deontological approach to ethics states a rule-based approach to ethics and outlines four principles. These principles sometimes overlap and there are occasions where they conflict.

- The principle of autonomy for children dictates that children's rights to make decisions regarding their own lives are respected. In research this means that children have free will to decide about participation.
- When adhering to the principle of justice researchers are obliged to ensure that prospective participants have equal rights of access to be involved and that particular groups are not exploited for the benefit of others.
- The principle of beneficence requires that the research has some benefits either to the participants directly, or child populations more broadly.
- The principle of non-maleficence indicates that involvement in your research will not have any iatrogenic impact. The child should not be harmed physically or psychologically by participating.

Autonomy

In the context of child mental health, professionals are likely to view autonomy from a developmental perspective in relation to the child's level of maturation and social/psychological development (Hoagwood et al., 1996; Paul et al., 2006). As a researcher you will need to respect the child's autonomy. In practice this means that you will need to ensure that you obtain the parent's and child's consent/assent to participate and to be certain that the child is able to exercise their right to withdraw if they wish.

Informed consent and the right to withdraw   When conducting research with children it will be essential in most cases to obtain consent from parents before you can approach children. In some circumstances, however, this can be problematic or even damaging to the research or participants (Geluda et al., 2005).

> ## Example
>
> You may be interested in the effects of having a termination of pregnancy on mental health in older girls. It may be the case, however, that these girls have not informed their parents of the termination. It may be advisable to consult with the ethics committee to discuss going ahead with the project without parental consent.

It is, however, expected that you will obtain consent from the children themselves, although there may be some exceptions. Often the age of the child is used as the benchmark for competency (Morrow & Richards, 1996). However, competency is also based on maturity, understanding and intelligence (Cocks, 2006). These factors constitute the legal framework of 'Gillick competency' which is used in the field of medicine in relation to children's treatment decisions.

There are three main components to informed consent: information is presented in an understandable way; consent is voluntary; and the participant has capacity to provide consent (Beresford, 1997). The Mental Capacity Act (Mental Health Foundation, 1999) stipulates that for an individual to demonstrate mental capacity to make a decision then the following criteria must be considered:

- Can the individual understand information given to them?
- Can the individual retain that information long enough to be able to make a decision?
- Can the individual weigh up the information available to make a decision?
- Can the individual communicate their decision to you?

These four criteria will be useful questions for you to ask when assessing the capacity of your potential participants to consent in your research.

> **!** You may not necessarily have the required skills to make a capacity assessment but it is important where required, that someone sufficiently qualified does this for you (Hunter & Pierscionek, 2007). A child however, may only be able to give assent (see below for definition and description).

If individuals do not fully understand the nature of the research they are not in a position to give informed consent (Oliver, 2010). Gaining clear informed consent from children, particularly younger children or those with limited competence, may not be feasible. Some researchers therefore prefer to obtain 'assent' from children (Alderson & Morrow, 2004). This is considered to be ethically acceptable providing parental consent is already in place. See Table 4.2.

Table 4.2   Consent

Level	Description
Consent	Consent is when the child actively communicates that he/she is willing to participate in the research and has capacity to do so.
Assent	Assent is when the child complies with or implies agreement to engage in the research.
Dissent	Dissent is when the child indicates that they do not want to participate. They may do this verbally or non-verbally.

When gaining consent from parents/children or assent you will need to ask them to sign a form that you will need to design. We provide an example of our 'assent' form in Figure 4.2.

The consent form should be accompanied by an information sheet so that the children/parents are fully aware of what is involved. When designing your information sheets it is important that you communicate the important information about the purpose of the study, the expectations of the participant, the risks and benefits, the time-frame, ethical principles, contact details and complaints procedure. All of these things need to be communicated in an age-appropriate format taking into consideration any other potential barriers to the participant's understanding. We give an example of a section (from page 2) of our information sheet in Figure 4.3 and then consider these key points in Table 4.3.

As we noted in Table 4.2 not all children will consent/assent, however dissent may not be overt but may be indicated subtly. You need to be attentive to non-verbal cues which may indicate dissent during the process of seeking informed consent/assent. Remember that consent is an iterative

Decision-making in child mental health assessments – V2 12/10/2010

University logo here

Assent form for young people
(To be completed by the child and their parent/guardian)

University address here
Name of organisation
Department
Address
Postcode

Centre number: Number here
Study number: 10/H0401/81

Family identification number:

Decision-making in child mental health assessments: Analysis of triage appointments in a child mental health service

Dr Michelle O'Reilly, *Colleagues names here*

Child (or if unable, parent on their behalf)/young person to circle all they agree with:

1. Has somebody explained this project to you?   Yes / No

2. Have you asked all the questions you want?   Yes / No

3. Do you understand it's OK to stop taking part at anytime?   Yes / No

4. Are you happy to take part?   Yes / No

If any answers are 'no' or you **do not** want to take part, **do not** sign your name!

If you **do** want to take part, you can **write your name** below

Your name   _____

Date   _____

The doctor who explained this project to you needs to sign too:

Print Name   _____

Sign   _____

Date   _____   Thank you

When completed: 1 for participant; 1 for researcher site file; 1 (original) to be kept in medical notes

Figure 4.2 Assent form

process and needs to be revisited throughout all stages of the research process, not just at the information giving stage (O'Reilly et al., 2011). If at any stage during data collection or later during debriefing children indicate signs of dissent or a desire to change their minds/withdraw from the study it is your responsibility to ensure that the child is free to exercise this right.

Information sheet for younger children–version 2 – 12/10/2010

Why have I been asked to take part?

We are asking all children and their families who attend the first appointment to take part. Every family is being asked if they would like to take part in the research project.

Did anyone else check the study is OK to do?

Before the research is allowed to happen, it has to be checked by a group of people called a Research Ethics Committee. They make sure the research is fair. Your project has been checked by the [name of ethics committee here].

Do I have to take part?

Taking part in the research is up to you.

We will ask you and your parents/carers if you want to take part but it is your choice if you want to.

If you do not, the appointment will not be videoed but everything else will remain the same.

What will happen to me if I take part in the research?

If you do take part in the research there will be nothing different from a normal appointment except the meeting will be videoed so researchers can look at it at a later time.

Only the first time you come will be videoed. If you come for further appointments we will not have to video them.

Will joining in with the study help me?

We cannot promise the study will help you but the information we gain might help treat other young people in the future.

Figure 4.3 Section of an information sheet

Table 4.3 Designing an information sheet for children

Information	Description
Purpose of the study	Communicate to the child what your study is about, why you are doing it and how it is important.
Expectations of the participant	Tell the child what they are agreeing to in terms of how much time they will be participating for, whether they will have to travel, who else is involved, and what they need to do for you.
Risks and benefits	Illustrate any benefits that the child may encounter from participating (such as rewards or inducements) and any risks that they may be exposed to (such as any emotional impact).
Time-frame	This relates to the time-frame of the project as well as the immediate time they will need to devote to you. You should communicate when they will be needed, when/if you might communicate the results/findings back to them.

(Continued)

Table 4.3 (Continued)

Information	Description
Ethical principles	It is essential that you outline all of the key ethical considerations to them. This includes their right to withdraw, where the data will be stored and how long for, confidentiality and anonymity. It should be clear here that their non-participation will not affect any routine care/treatments they are being provided with.
Contact details and complaints	It is helpful to provide as many ways of contacting you as possible, such as email, mobile (cell) phone, landline, post. It may not be advisable to provide personal contact details, however, use work contacts where possible. It is important that you outline the complaints procedure.

Possible scenario = You are interviewing a child with diagnosed bulimia about her experiences of a particular intervention. Approximately half way through the interview you notice that she keeps checking her watch and looking at the door. Her answers to your questions are getting shorter and there are subtle signs of agitation.

Possible solution = It is fairly clear that this child no longer wants to continue the interview and you should provide her with the option to stop. You need to be clear whether she is happy to allow you to keep the data she has or whether she has changed her mind and no longer wants to be part of your project. You might also want to find out the reason for the behaviour as she may be happy to continue the rest of the interview another day.

Justice

The principle of justice relates to the notion of equality, in terms of access to research participation and protection from exploitation. In child mental health this is especially important given that these children constitute a vulnerable population. This has tended to result in a more paternalistic position being adopted by researchers and ethics committees which seek to protect children in research. This illuminates a tension between the principle of autonomy and the paternalistic element of the principle of justice.

Power and coercion/inducement   An important issue in conducting mental health research is the need to avoid coercing individuals into participation by recognising the position of power that you are in (Davies, 2005). We discussed this earlier in Chapter 3 where we noted that in your professional role you may inadvertently coerce the child to participate. Power is not a fixed concept, rather it is fluid and shifting (Christensen, 2004).

In conducting mental health research with children there is interplay of all of the potential asymmetries as described previously in Chapter 3: adult/child, researcher/participant, health advantage/disadvantage and practitioner/patient (client/pupil). Additionally one of the consequences of experiencing mental health difficulties is that there is often a stigma attached which can have both social and economic consequences as well as a subjective impact on the sense of self (Davies, 2005). The link between social disadvantage and the development of mental health difficulties is well established (Meltzer et al., 2004). Conversely having a child with mental health difficulties can put economic strain on the family (Busch & Barry, 2007).

Research indicates that there are two key factors affecting willingness to participate: risk and monetary compensation (Dunn et al., 2009). Offering participants payment for their involvement in research is a form of inducement. However, an ethical concern for vulnerable families is that financial inducements may unduly influence participants to participate (Bagley et al., 2007). There is thus an argument that inducement can compromise informed consent as participants may not fully consider the risks (Grady, 2005), or they may not be well able to judge those risks in advance (McNeill, 1997). This has become an ethical concern as payment is sometimes perceived as a form of coercion. Coercion involves the deliberate imposition of one person's will over another and usually takes the form of threats (Wilkinson & Moore, 1997). If inducement were to become coercion, this would risk an infringement of the justice principle in relation to the elevated susceptibility of these families. However, inducements in the form of financial reward/compensation are not usually threats (Wilkinson & Moore 1997) and therefore may be ethically acceptable mechanisms for increasing participant involvement. However, it should be noted therefore that inducement has the potential to expose participants to risks that they may not otherwise take without the financial payment (McNeill, 1997).

 Offering payment may attract more vulnerable lower socio-economic status groups (Grady, 2005) which may bias your sample.

Possible scenario = You are running focus groups with young people who participate in mental health services due to drug or alcohol abuse. You want to run 5 groups each with 5–6 participants but you are having trouble recruiting. You have a small budget so you decide to offer £20 inducement. After you have advertised this you suddenly find lots of young people volunteering. You are now concerned that they may spend the money on substances.

(Continued)

(Continued)

Possible solution = There are different ways you could handle this. First you may want to question whether interviews might be a better method. It could be that the young people did not want to discuss their problems in front of others. Alternatively you could have offered a different type of incentive, a gift card or book token. Another possibility would be to build better relationships with gatekeepers and allow them to facilitate your recruitment drive.

Beneficence and non-maleficence

Beneficence refers to the ethical obligation to ensure that your research is of benefit either to the child directly or children and families generally. Research inevitably involves some risk and/or inconvenience to participants and you have an obligation to weigh this against any potential benefits of your research. On an individual level benefit may be the receipt of an incentive or appreciation. As we discussed earlier this has the potential to infringe the principle of justice, but may actually be of some benefit to the participants. The research, however, may not be of direct benefit to the individual participants but the purpose of conducting research is to gain knowledge which can be used to inform services and practitioners. It is therefore vital within the principle of beneficence that you think carefully about how you will disseminate your findings.

Non-maleficence relates to the risks of the project and is an ethical guiding principle which dictates that you ensure you protect your participants from harm. Whilst beneficence and non-maleficence have some overlap with autonomy and justice, there are mechanisms you can employ to reduce the risks and increase benefits.

Of particular importance for research with child participants is confidentiality and anonymity. It is more likely that children rather than adults may impulsively disclose private aspects of their lives and establish trust with a stranger more readily (Singh & Keenan, 2010). This is especially problematic in qualitative research as there is also a risk of betrayal which arises in part from the greater closeness that may develop between the participant and researcher (Shaw, 2008).

Anonymity and confidentiality

Anonymity refers to the removal of all features that may identify the children in any representations of the data. This means you must replace names with pseudonyms/numbers and take out any identifying characteristics such as locations, friends, family or pets' names. Children do have a reasonable understanding of the notion of anonymity and have mixed views about it (O'Reilly, Karim, et al., 2012). Interestingly, participants often have strong views about which pseudonyms they prefer (Corden & Sainsbury, 2006) and sometimes prefer to be offered the choice to have their real names used (Giordano et al., 2007).

Anonymity is one way of ensuring confidentiality of participants. Confidentiality relates to assuring privacy to participants and protecting the raw data. It also refers to maintaining professional integrity relating to not discussing personal details with colleagues and friends outside of the research team. Qualitative health research particularly collects a significant volume of personal and sensitive information (Richards & Schwartz, 2002) and confidentiality is utilised as a mechanism to protect participants from harm. Confidentiality and anonymity should be considered on the information sheet and we show the section from our parental information sheet in Figure 4.4.

Children therefore remain 'safer' in research as confidentiality has potential to reduce their vulnerability (Giordano et al., 2007). This is because vulnerable populations may face harmful consequences if their identities or personal details are revealed (Baez, 2002). Although you may take every care to protect the identity of the children in your research by anonymising the transcript, the richness of qualitative data can sometimes mean that there is a risk of deductive disclosure. Deductive disclosure refers to details in the transcript being recognisable to other people known to the research participants (Sieber, 1992).

Will my taking part in the study be kept confidential?

Data will be collected through the use of video-recording equipment. Your normal triage session will be recorded and the tape passed to the research team. Care will be taken during this process. This tape will be transcribed and then securely stored in a locked, reinforced cupboard at the Greenwood Institute. The transcripts will be anonymous and all identifying features removed from them. If the research team show any clips from the video to professionals outside of the research team, faces will be obscured with pixels and names removed. For example if used for other research or meetings.

What will happen to the results of the research study?

The data provided will be subjected to language-based analyses and disseminated through research reports and published academic papers. In this process all of your identifying features will be removed from your quotations to maintain confidentiality and anonymity.

Figure 4.4   Confidentiality and the parent information sheet

> ❗ By removing and changing the identifying features there is a risk that the meaning of the stories may be altered (Kaiser, 2009).

Possible scenario = You have been collecting diary entries from children about the emotional effects of being diagnosed with cancer. Each child has been keeping a log of their feelings associated with particular aspects of their daily lives including hospital visits and going to school. Many of the children are from the same region and therefore when you present your workshop for teachers you are concerned that as local members they may recognise the children from some of the unique experiences noted down.

Possible solutions = This is a tricky issue but some experiences will be clearly more identifying than others and should not be included in your workshop presentation. Where possible reveal little about the location from which the children were recruited. You may also want to consult with the children themselves. You may also decide not to present to teachers from that geographical area if this is too contentious.

Safeguarding

If a child does reveal something concerning then you will need to consider breaking the confidentiality agreement in order to safeguard their well-being. Child mental health research has an increased possibility that evidence of problems, illegal behaviour, health-compromising behaviours or health problems unknown to adults may be discussed (Fisher et al., 2002). Additionally there is a possibility that incidences of abuse may be uncovered. This is an important issue when researching children and not an easy one to navigate. If you are doing research with a child there is a possibility they may reveal something which implies risk to their safety, but you do need to be careful that you are cautious in any interpretations you make (Cameron, 2005).

If you have a clinical role your professional responsibility for safeguarding may be clear as there are guidelines for medicine and education which outline the obligations of professionals (Williamson et al., 2005). Your obligations as a researcher may, however, be less clear, especially given the promised confidentiality to your participants.

Possible scenario = During an interview with a child about their experiences of taking medication the child tells you that they do not like it when their uncle brings them their medication as he hurts them. You try to find out more but the child does not provide you with further information.

Possible solutions =

- Safeguarding issues should always form a part of the protocol design.
- Be aware of the local safeguarding procedures.
- Outline clearly any limits to confidentiality to parents and children before you start data collection.
- Consult with other members of the research team or your supervisor (both if possible) to establish the course of action.

Debriefing

Fortunately most child mental health research goes smoothly without raising any issues for safeguarding and without the need to break promises of confidentiality. This does not necessarily guarantee that you have done no psychological harm to the child though and you need to ensure that the child is comfortable when they leave you. One mechanism for checking this is through debriefing. This usually occurs at the end of a particular data collection aspect of your research and ensures that the child leaves the research in a similar physical and emotional state as they arrived.

Possible scenario = You have been interviewing a child about the effects of their speech impairment in the classroom at school. During the interview the child tells you about bullying and gets upset. You understand that the teachers and parents are both aware of this problem, but your immediate concern is the child's distress as they are crying in the interview.

Possible solution = Due to the child's distress, it is best to stop the recording and allow the child a break. You could give the child a tissue and you would offer to bring the parent back into the room if available. It is best not to offer physical comfort. If the child becomes calmer you can ask if they wish to continue the interview and they must be given every opportunity to withdraw. At the end you need to debrief and make sure that they are no longer distressed. Take time to talk to the child and check they are feeling better. You might want to ask if it is okay to share with the parent so that the parent is aware.

Summary

This chapter has outlined the importance of using an ethical framework when engaging in research with children who have mental health difficulties. The reasons why ethics are important in this kind of research have been illuminated with some indications regarding why these matter particularly for child participants. In this chapter we have introduced you to the role of ethics committees and provided you with some practical tips for managing review. This is done alongside caution that ethics are iterative and do not stop with the ethics committee. We have paid particular attention to the specific ethical principles and the safeguarding children practices that are likely to be relevant to any child mental health project.

Key messages

- Applying an ethical framework is important to protect children in research.
- Ethical governance and committees can facilitate the ethicality of your research.
- The four key principles are: respect for autonomy, justice, beneficence and non-maleficence.

Further reading

DuBois, J. (2008). *Ethics in mental health research: principles, guidance, and cases.* Oxford: Oxford University Press.

Hoagwood, K., Jensen, P. & Fisher, C. (eds) (1996). *Ethical issues in mental health research with children and adolescents.* New Jersey: Lawrence Earlbaum Associates.

Oliver, P. (2010). *The student's guide to research ethics* (Second edition). Berkshire: Open University Press.

PART TWO
GETTING STARTED

CHAPTER 5

PLANNING A CHILD-FOCUSED PROJECT

Learning outcomes

- Choose an appropriate topic of study.
- Develop a child relevant research question.
- Construct a proposal.
- Keep a research diary.
- Critically appreciate the importance of involving stakeholders/service users.
- Undertake a pilot study.

Introduction

For your project to be successful it is important that you plan it effectively. To do this it is necessary to think about several issues and perform some important tasks. Obviously you need to think about which area of child mental health you are interested in researching, narrowing down your focus can be challenging, however. In this chapter we provide a toolkit for choosing a worthy topic of research and provide you with practical strategies for turning this into a strong research question. Once the initial stages are complete you need to define your research in a more developed way by generating a proposal/protocol. There are different styles of presenting these and in this chapter we offer you some advice on how to develop one that is convincing and informative. We also provide information on involving stakeholders and service users throughout the process and illustrate the importance of maintaining a research diary. The chapter concludes with some practical guidance regarding conducting a pilot study and alerts you to some of the pitfalls of poor planning.

Avoiding poor planning

This chapter is designed to help you with your planning and avoid some of the common mistakes that are often made by those new to qualitative research. Before we go through the key elements of planning we first introduce you to some of the pitfalls and consequences of poor planning so that you can bear these in mind as you read through the chapter:

- A poorly defined research question is likely to mean that you lose focus and direction.
- The research question informs the methodology and methods, so you should avoid starting with method and trying to generate a question that fits it.
- You should be aware of your theoretical position before you start as this will shape your decisions.
- A poorly written research proposal is likely to result in a poorly conducted piece of research.
- You need to pilot your method as you do not want to find the imperfections or mistakes during your actual data collection.
- Failing to keep a research diary will mean that you find it difficult to be reflexive throughout the process or transparent in your dissemination.

Choosing a topic

It is suggested that research should always be driven by curiosity (White, 2009) and your own curiosity is a good place to start. The topic that you choose to study in your research project will be informed by several factors. The first is likely to be the environment or context in which you are studying or working.

> **Example**
>
> If you are working in an eating disorders clinic this might inform your research interest in this area.

The second is potentially any personal or professional experience you have in an area.

> **Example**
>
> You may have a niece or other relative who has experienced anorexia nervosa which prompts your interest in this area.

The third is personal interest in an area of child mental health, stemming from literature you have read, or ideas promoted by your supervisor (clinical or academic).

> **Example**
>
> A work colleague has already published some research on bulimia in South Asian girls and you are interested in taking this further.

We illustrate this funnelling of ideas in Figure 5.1.

Once you have established the topic area the next step is to refine your ideas. This can be achieved through two parallel processes: brainstorming and reading. At this stage some ideas will be discounted because they have already been researched extensively and others may not be possible practically with the time and resources you have. Remaining ideas can be refined through discussions with colleagues.

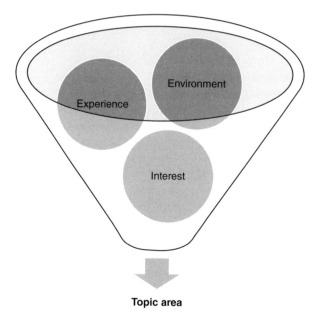

Figure 5.1   Generating a research topic

> **!** Caution: Resist the temptation to try to do too much in one project. It is important to narrow down your focus.

Your views of children

Your views about children are important. This has been a long-debated topic, with new perspectives viewing childhood as historically, politically and culturally influenced, as well as dynamic and changing. This means that children are now seen as a distinct population with views and rights (Corsaro, 2011). The shifting views on childhood have affected the way we conduct research with children. Children participating in research have been conceptualised in many ways and Alderson (2005) lists seven views:

1. The child as innocent and needing protection.
2. The child as deprived or disadvantaged and needing resources.
3. The child as criminal and needing control.
4. The child as ignorant and requiring education.
5. The child as excluded and needing special opportunities.
6. The child as disabled and a victim of a rejecting society.
7. The child as resourceful.

These changes have meant that we have moved away from doing research *'on'* children to doing research *'with'* them. In research terms therefore, children have been viewed in three ways as described by Punch (2002):

- First is an approach which considers children to be practically the same as adults and therefore uses the same methods to study them.
- Second is an approach which perceives children as different from adults and uses participant observation or ethnography to examine the world of the child.
- Third is an approach which understands children as similar to adults but with different competencies and there are a range of innovative and adapted techniques.

When you build your research question it is important you reflect on your views of children and consider how they shape your research. For example, do you think of children as miniature adults or do you see them as growing individuals different from adults? Do you believe that children have the right to make their own decisions or that adults should make decisions for them?

How to develop a research question

If you are going to undertake qualitative research then you will need a good research question. This is quite difficult to do well and we provide you with a model to help you consider the process in practice.

 Do not underestimate how long it will take you to develop a good research question (White, 2009).

The best way to develop your question is to brainstorm ideas and write down everything that interests you or comes to mind. You will of course need to organise your thinking before you turn those ideas into a question and we have devised a useful way of thinking about research questions using the acronym 'STEPS'.

Specific	A narrow field of study	
		---------------HOW skills
Timely	An achievable time-frame and contemporary project	
Enquiry	What kind of question	
Participants	Who is being studied	---------------WHAT skills
Subject	The topic of interest	

While STEPS is not prescriptive, it is a good way to think about how to write a question. When thinking about the three key 'WHAT' ingredients of a good research question: enquiry, participants and subject, it is important to apply the first two 'HOW' skills, specific and timely, to each of these 'ingredients'.

The following examples are provided to demonstrate this STEPS model and how it can be used for your own research project.

Example 1

How do Indian boys experience eating disorder interventions in British inpatient settings?

Example 2

What reasons do anorexic girls provide for their initial restrictive eating behaviours?

Enquiry relates to the nature of the question. In qualitative research this is usually represented as 'what', 'how' or 'why'. These are typically words which open the question and determine its direction. In Example 1, the word 'how' is used to indicate the direction that the question is taking and explicates the type of question it is. The focus of Example 2 is on the nature of the reasons and asks a 'what' prefaced question. Remember that qualitative research questions need to be open (not closed) questions.

Participants relates to the group of individuals being studied. The demographic characteristics of your participants are usefully defined within the question. In Example 1 the participant group is 'Indian boys' whereas in Example 2 the focus is on 'anorexic girls'.

Subject relates to the topic of the research. This again needs to be specific and clear. This part of the question illustrates the main focus of the research. The subject specificity in Example 1 is that the question goes beyond eating disorder interventions generically to examine interventions carried out in inpatient settings. In Example 2 the subject is restrictive eating patterns which initially preceded the onset of the eating disorder.

Once you have designed your research question using these three 'ingredients' it is important to check that the question is specific and timely. This means that the question should be focused and should be contemporary and achievable in the time-frame.

A **Activity   Research question design**

Apply the STEPS model to each of the six questions below to determine their strengths and weaknesses.

1 Do girls eat more than boys?
2 How do younger children with suspected autism interact with adult caregivers in child mental health assessments?
3 What do girls from traveller communities give as explanations for their self-harming behaviours?
4 Can children learn to manage their depression?
5 Why don't children take their prescribed psychiatric medication even though both the psychiatrist and their parents have told them that they need to do this?
6 How do older children with early onset psychosis perceive the effects of the condition on their peer relationships?

You have hopefully identified questions 1, 4 and 5 as poorer examples while 2, 3 and 6 follow the STEPS model. Questions 1 and 4 are more quantitative in nature as they seek to measure certain elements and are closed questions in their design. Question 5 is rather long and unwieldy; it has little focus and is not specific. Questions 2, 3 and 6 are open questions with a clear enquiry aspect to them. The participants in these questions are specifically defined and the subject clear. These three questions are also timely in that they address contemporary child mental health issues and should be achievable in a reasonable time-frame.

Additionally it is essential that your research question is ethical. We considered ethics in the previous chapter and you will need to consider those issues as you develop and refine your research question. This is especially important in the area of mental health. DuBois (2008) noted four core issues:

1. Some mental health research has contributed to the stigma of conditions in particular groups by highlighting greater prevalence in minority groups.
2. Some research questions fail to reflect the priorities of consumers.
3. Some research questions are motivated by profit and while not inherently unethical per se should be scrutinised carefully.
4. Some research questions are unethical due to the fact that they will not generate knowledge, rather are likely to reinforce the assumptions upon which they rest.

Inclusion/exclusion criteria

To define the participants section of the research question you need to be quite specific about your inclusion and exclusion criteria. Inclusion criteria are those markers which you specify must be present in your participant sample. These are the characteristics the participants must have if they are to be included in your research so you can address your aims and objectives.

Example

If you are looking at the eating patterns of children with OCD you will need to include children with a formal diagnosis of the condition and you may decide to only include children who have not had treatment, or of a particular age group.

Exclusion criteria are markers to exclude individuals from your study. These are criteria that disqualify possible participants from involvement. These criteria need to be as clearly defined as possible in order to facilitate the process of recruitment and data collection.

Example

If you are looking at the eating patterns of children with OCD, you may choose to exclude those with eating disorders or particular intolerances, such as nut allergies.

Developing a proposal/protocol

A research proposal is a document which outlines the theoretical and practical aspects of your planned project. It is written at the beginning of the process to help you plan your research. Although it may seem obvious to you that child mental health research is both necessary and important, you will need to convey this to several audiences.

 Do not be tempted to think that writing a proposal is merely a formality, it is a useful exercise to help others judge the quality of your work (Robson, 2011).

Table 5.1   Possible audiences

Audiences	
Funding bodies	You may be trying to acquire money to help you carry out your project.
Ethics committees	It is fairly typical for ethics committees to request a copy of the proposal to help them contextualise the ethical sensitivities of your project.
Educational institutions	A common audience is the educational institution, particularly if carried out as part of a formal qualification.
Other members of the research team	If you are working on a project as part of a team they will be guided by the proposal that you develop as this will illustrate key decisions being made.
Yourself	Do not underestimate how important the proposal will be to you. It will provide you with a platform for your reading and any decisions you make.

It may be that you are writing your proposal for more than one audience and you may need to produce slightly different versions of it. We indicate some of the possible audiences in Table 5.1.

One audience is the funding body and the purpose is to illustrate the value of your ideas to acquire finances. Applying for funding is competitive and it can be challenging to convince funding bodies that your research is worthy of investment. The purpose of a proposal for this audience is to illuminate the value of your project and show that your research is important. Even if you are not applying for money, when you write your proposal it is helpful to think of your work in this way when considering the rationale. Ask yourself the question '*is this research worth funding*?' Think about whether children or families might benefit from it and what contribution you are making to the field of child mental health. Remember that some indication of any potential outputs from your study will be helpful (Eve, 2008).

 Your study should have some value and you should be able to provide a rationale for the need for it.

If you are undertaking your research as part of an educational qualification then your proposal will probably be judged by your supervisor and your examiners. The proposal will help your supervisor to:

- Judge the feasibility of your research.
- Assess the quality of your writing.
- Appreciate the value of your project.

It is possible that the proposal will be formally assessed, making up a percentage of your overall achievement. Alternatively it may form part of the appendices of your thesis/dissertation and will be looked at by the examiners to understand your decision-making process. This means that your proposal has a lot of work to do to convince the audiences that your research is useful and shows that you have thought about all of the procedural and ethical elements.

How to write a proposal

The first point to remember when you begin drafting your proposal is that different institutions have different templates, signposts and word lengths. Think about the audience you are writing for as they may have specific expectations regarding what your proposal should deliver.

 It is essential that you use the guidelines of the educational institution or funding body to help you shape your proposal and use the suggested headings they provide.

Despite these differences there are a number of features which are likely to be expected.

Title page

The title page should illustrate the exact title of your project. This should reflect the area of child mental health that you are planning to study and should be original and eye-catching.

 Do not think of your title as fixed once you have used it in your proposal. You may find that it will need to be revised as your research unfolds.

Introduction/literature review

This part of the proposal is the first part that your reader evaluates and it sets the context for your research. The introduction is not a literature review in a conventional sense but does function to show the reader how your child mental health research fits with the broader evidence (Punch, 2000). When developing the introduction it is important to remember that it forms part of the argument as to why your research is needed. Start broadly with a critical appraisal of the general evidence and narrow your discussion down to lead to the point of your work. As you develop your discussion using the published research you should be helping the reader to appreciate a particular gap in knowledge, which you are proposing to fill. This section of the proposal gives you an opportunity to impress the reader with your commitment and professionalism (Robson, 2011).

When you have contextualised where your research project fits within the broader evidence-base it is important that you clearly state your research question. This may consist of a singular broad research question or it may have sub-questions attached to it.

Aims and rationale

In this section you provide a rationale by illuminating how your aims and objectives will address the research question that you have offered. Show the reader how you will fill that gap in knowledge and why. Remember that a research aim is different to an objective.

> ### Example
>
> Your research may <u>aim</u> to elicit the perceptions of refugee children's experiences of bereavement with an <u>objective</u> of producing a simple information leaflet for childhood bereavement services to give out.

> ### Example
>
> Your research may <u>aim</u> to recognise the experiences of children in drug and alcohol services with an <u>objective</u> of providing training courses for mental health professionals who work with these groups.

Aims and objectives can be difficult to summarise but try to be as succinct as possible. It should be a clear and concise part of the proposal. You may find it useful to write out your aims as questions in the first instance and then transform them into actual aims (Eve, 2008).

Approach and method

This is an important element of the proposal which provides your reader with decisions regarding the design of your project. You should provide a clear rationale here as to why a qualitative approach is appropriate with a clear strategy for addressing your research question to meet your aims and objectives. It is important that you are familiar with the benefits and limitations of using your chosen approach to study the particular aspect of child mental health. If you are doing qualitative work then you need to be clear about any theoretical assumptions being made (Eve, 2008). In this section you need to show the reader which methods you are going to use for your research. This should include a rationale for the methods of data collection and analysis as well as any information about other important processes such as recording and transcription.

Access and ethics

In this section you will need to provide details about your recruitment strategy, including information on sampling. You need to provide some contextual detail for your reader regarding the demographics of your sample, your sampling strategy, potential gatekeepers and any pilot work undertaken. It is important that you are clear how many children, families or professionals will be recruited and what your inclusion/exclusion criteria are.

Outline any ethical concerns and indicate the strategies you will employ to address those sensitivities. Your discipline should have its own research ethical code of practice and this should be clearly stated. Additionally your work is likely to be reviewed by an ethics committee and you should show which one will be reviewing your work.

Expected contribution

A useful signpost can be the expected contribution of your research. This section allows you to show how your project has value to other children, their families, mental health professionals or society more generally. This is your opportunity to demonstrate how your research may have the potential to inform policy or form part of the evidence-base drawn upon to develop legislation. This part of the proposal can demonstrate the level of practical applicability for your research and in doing so highlight the contribution your research will make.

Timescale

You should have thought about the time-frame for completing your project. If you are undertaking your research as part of an educational qualification your time-frame may be quite short. However long you have to develop and implement your ideas it is necessary to highlight these in your research proposal. It is important that these are realistic, achievable and sensible, bearing in mind that there may be unanticipated difficulties along the way.

Dissemination

It is helpful to indicate how your work will be disseminated and to whom. You may want to publish your findings in peer-reviewed journals and present it at conferences. You may want to provide informative reports to specific service user groups or families. Alternatively you may disseminate through your educational qualification in the form of your thesis/dissertation.

Budget

This will depend on the purpose of your proposal and intended audience but it can be helpful to break down the costs of your research. You may have to factor in travel costs and there are also costs associated with purchasing recording equipment and carrying out transcription. It is necessary to be honest about the overall costs of your research and be precise, especially if you are applying for funding.

Final drafts

Once you have drafted your proposal it is advisable to get some advice. If you have an academic/clinical supervisor they may be able to provide you with feedback regarding the quality of your writing. It is important that you do not submit your proposal without having it checked by someone else or without proof reading it first. The previous section provided some of the likely signposts to use in your proposal but as we mentioned earlier it is important that you consult the guidelines you are provided with. There are lots of things you can do to make your proposal more attractive and appealing and we provide you with some general tips in Table 5.2.

The research diary

Given the sensitive nature of child mental health and the vulnerability of participants it is essential that you keep a research diary. This diary should provide a chronological account of the events, decisions and questions occurring throughout the project (Burgess, 1981). This may feel tedious at first but you will start to see the benefits of keeping your diary up-to-date

Table 5.2 Tips for proposals

	Tips
Timescale	Remember to illustrate that you have been mindful of factors which may influence your timescale. For example children's school holidays may hinder/facilitate your access depending on your route for recruitment.
Terminology	Be mindful of the language you use. Acceptable terms are changing and you need to make sure your proposal is politically correct.
Word limits	Remember that word limits are imposed for a reason. Make sure that you stick to the agreed length.
Reading	Your audience will expect you to have read well. This reading should include information about topic, methods and ethics.
Structure	Make sure the order in which you signpost the different sections of your proposal is logical and sensible. This should enable you to formulate a clear argument throughout, reaching the conclusion that your research has value and is needed.
Respect	Remember that despite many advances mental health difficulties are still relatively stigmatised and you need to demonstrate that you will treat your participants with respect.

as you make progress. There are lots of different modalities for keeping a diary but the most common include:

- Lap-top/computer/tablet records – keeping an electronic folder of documents which track your project progress and process.
- Large paper notebook – traditional pen and paper method can be useful. Some notebooks come with dividers so that you can separate or categorise your diary entries.
- A calendar style diary – some prefer to have an actual diary with dates so that they can record key points on each day of the week. A day-per-view diary is preferable in this case.

Keeping a research diary is important for many reasons. These include making your reasoning transparent (Silverman, 2009), providing a clear audit trail (Smith, 1999), aiding reflection (Nadin & Cassell, 2006), tracking appointments/events (Blaxter et al., 2001) and facilitating time management (Silverman, 2009). There are, therefore, three main purposes to keeping a research diary:

- *To record factual information* – including references, dates of events, appointments and participant demographics.
- *To be reflective* – a component which is especially important in qualitative research as reflexivity requires awareness and consideration of your personal reactions to events and data collection. This is an opportunity to write down your thoughts and feelings as they occur.
- *To record decisions made throughout the process* – including how and why particular methods were chosen, why certain participants were included/excluded and why any changes to the proposal were made.

> ## *A*   Activity   Start your diary
>
> Now is as good a time as any to start your research diary. Make a decision regarding whether you are going to keep it electronically or on paper and write your first entry now. Give it a title, something like 'my feelings at the start of the process' and under that heading write a couple of sentences about how you feel right now in terms of planning your research project.

Facts

A key purpose of the research diary is to record factual information. Some of this will be generated from your reading, some from discussing your project with others and some from communicating with participants. It is important to keep a record of any appointments or events attended, when you attended them, why you attended them and what happened. You can also keep a record of any reading, literature search terms you have employed or any other sources of information utilised.

> ## Example   Facts
>
> I attended a workshop today as part of my training through work on the use of CBT for children with OCD. This was a really useful workshop and the leader gave me her contact details as she is interested in my project. Her email address is SS3y@dd.com[1]. I intend to email her tomorrow as she recommended a good book.

This example illustrates one of the useful ways in which factual information can be recorded. By having people's contact details or dates of events recorded you will know exactly where to find them when you need them.

Reflection/reflexivity

If you are familiar with clinical practice then you should have some understanding of the importance of reflection. Researching children can involve dealing with sensitive or emotive topics and one useful way of managing this is to write it down. Reflecting on your characteristics, your personality and who you are as a person, as well as documenting the ways in which

---

[1]Fictional email

different elements of the research process affect you, will provide you with some useful information for writing later. This process of reflection also helps to promote the trustworthiness of the data and integrity of the process which is part of ensuring quality in qualitative work (Nadin & Cassell, 2006).

Example   Reflections

I interviewed a child's father today[2] and he was really arrogant. I struggled to keep my focus in the interview. He was critical of the mother for taking his child to the mental health service as he denies that there is a problem. His daughter has been diagnosed with anorexia but he claims that she is just a picky eater, going through a phase. He doesn't see the point in her having therapy for it and says she is attention-seeking. He included me in that statement. I haven't been involved in his daughter's care. Think I feel quite cross about it.

Being reflective in a diary can give you an opportunity to highlight how you feel about something. You can challenge your own thoughts as well as write down what happened. Over a series of reflective entries you may start to see patterns emerging and these can be discussed with your peers, colleagues or supervisors. We return to the issue of reflexivity later in the book.

Decision-making

When you come to disseminate it will become necessary to provide information on some of the decisions you made. Memory can be unreliable and it is important not to rely on your ability to recall decisions. Instead it is helpful to write a brief note in your diary about what the decision was, why you made it, what evidence you used to make it, who you consulted during that decision-making process and any related outcomes of that decision.

Example   Decision-making

Following supervision I have decided to narrow down the focus of my project[3]. My supervisor and I agreed that including children from all age groups to explore the experiences of psychosis was misguided as

---

[2]Fictional example

[3]Fictional example

this is a mental health difficulty that does not tend to occur in younger children. I have decided to include older children only in my study. I have found two research articles which talk about the average onset age and I will include these as evidence for my decision.

This example illustrates how choices made early on may need to be changed once you have consulted others and read more about the subject. No matter how small or large the decisions, it is essential that you document them in some way in the research diary. You will be pleased that you did this later on in the process.

Involving stakeholders or service-users

There are many reasons why researchers find it valuable to consult stakeholders and service-users during research. In the UK, the Department of Health (1999) advocates that the involvement of service-users is imperative in clinical research because they have additional skills and experiences which complement those of the researcher (Goodare & Lockwood, 1999).

A best-practice model advocates a stakeholder group consisting of several adults with an interest in the broad topic and project aims. This group should be consulted by the researcher throughout the research process and is particularly important during the design stage where key decisions are made. This is complemented by the service-user group which consists of a number of children/parents who have the expertise to help guide the project and refine areas that are ambiguous or open to misinterpretation.

Example

We use the research question from earlier in the chapter – How do Indian boys experience eating disorder interventions in British inpatient settings?

Stakeholder group: An ideal group would include a representative from the professional group who refer children to inpatient care (such as GPs), two or three members of inpatient teams who are involved in delivering interventions, (psychiatrists, other professionals), a local Indian community leader, parent representatives of eating-disordered Indian boys, a service manager and a social worker.

(Continued)

> *(Continued)*
>
> **Service-user group** – An ideal group would consist of a number of boys who have experienced an eating disorder of different ages, preferably those who have been in inpatient care, but might include girls, or those treated in outpatients.

Bringing together a stakeholder or service-user group can be challenging and it is unlikely that you will be able to have all members represented in your group. However, the example above gives a guide to who might be useful to have involved.

Service-user/stakeholder involvement should not be tokenistic but should positively influence the content of the research and make it more relevant to practice (Trivedi & Wykes, 2002). When conducting research with children, service-user consultation can be particularly helpful in translating adult-driven agendas into child-friendly language. It is important to develop partnerships with children who can provide you with insight into their worlds and ensure that their priorities are considered throughout your research. This is particularly important in qualitative research with children because meanings can vary between adults and children and discussion may prevent misunderstandings (Clark, 2005).

Conducting a pilot study

It is important that you conduct a pilot study before you start your research. This is so that you can get feedback from children relevant to your study and possibly their parents or other interested professionals. Pilot studies raise several fundamental issues related to the process and can help researchers learn lessons about research practice (Teijlingen et al., 2001). If you do not conduct a pilot study you risk being overwhelmed when the real research begins. Your lack of preparation may reduce the quality of your final research project and can impact on your dissemination (Sampson, 2004).

Table 5.3 provides some of the key benefits to conducting a pilot study for a child mental health project.

You can see from this table that there are many advantages to conducting a pilot study. By undertaking this phase you will be able to assess whether children are actually willing to engage with you in the research, why this is the case and any potential resistance to your work (Teijlingen et al., 2001). It is important during planning that you build in time to undertake a pilot study, but be careful not to underestimate how long they take. Pilot studies can vary in length, depth and intensity and the choices you make will relate to what purpose the pilot study has for you.

Table 5.3 Benefits of a pilot study

	Benefits
Access	• Allows you to build up relationships with gatekeepers. They may also help you to recruit other gatekeepers or provide you with information which is helpful during recruitment. • Allows you to develop your communication strategies and tests different methods, especially important with children or those with communication difficulties. • Affords you an opportunity to build interest amongst parents and professionals.
Ethics	• Allows you to test your informed consent procedures. • Allows you to check that children are actually reading the information sheets and to identify any barriers. • Provides you with a mechanism for checking that children understand the ethical concepts. • Provides an opportunity for undertaking a risk assessment to protect your own safety.
Materials	• Allows you to review the ethics documentation and make any necessary changes.
Data collection	• Allows you to check the practical aspects of your data collection technique. • Gives you an opportunity to obtain feedback from your pilot participants regarding how to improve it. • Allows you to check the value of and best use of any participatory techniques (such as use of photos or drawing).
Feasibility	• Informs the main project. • Allows you to identify any pitfalls or unanticipated barriers/problems. • You can use the information to convince others that the project is feasible.

 Make sure that you allow sufficient time to undertake your pilot study properly.

Some people will undertake a large pilot phase with several participants to inform the design of the project, whereas others will recruit a small number to test out a few of the important challenges, see our example below.

Personal case example: Pilot study

When designing one of our research projects about autism and psycho-education we felt that a pilot study was essential. Our area of interest was to get a better understanding of the information needs parents may have when their child is diagnosed with autism. We decided to interview parents. We wanted to be sure we were asking the right kinds of questions to be able to answer our research question: '*What information needs do parents of autistic children believe they have?*' There were two main aims:

1. To ascertain parental/carer experiences of current psycho-education.
2. To yield opinions on the form and structure of a web-based resource.

We decided to carry out a pilot study with two parents. This was so that we could practice interviewing as a methodological technique, test out the suitability of the interview questions, test the ethicality of our work and gain feedback from these parents to ensure that we had covered all important areas. Our pilot study identified four key issues:

1. *The interview schedule*: The responses from some of the pilot participants helped to identify some new and interesting questions that had not been thought of in the design stage. Additionally the pilot phase helped the researcher to familiarise herself with the schedule and become more comfortable asking questions.
2. *Expectations*: The pilot stage allowed the researcher to develop her interviewing skills. It allowed her to understand what to expect from participants and which prompts worked best.
3. *Time*: The pilot study gave some indication of roughly how long it took to go through the schedule and how long the interview would last.
4. *Environment*: Doing the pilot interviews made the researcher more aware of ways to put the participants at ease and illustrated the importance of building rapport. It made the researcher more aware of the physical environment and the importance of comfortable chairs and good lighting.

 Remember to include the findings and lessons learned from the pilot study when you write up your project later on.

Summary

In this chapter we have provided a framework for how to refine a topic area and develop a research question using the STEPS model. We have demonstrated how to write a research proposal based on an evaluation of the published literature and how this project will add to the current knowledge base. We have provided examples of how a research diary can be used throughout the planning and design stage of a research project in order to facilitate reflection and decision-making. Decision-making is an important element at all stages of the research and one that is enhanced by developing partnerships with service users and stakeholders. Finally the chapter considered the value of testing the design through a pilot study and provided some guidance on how to do this.

Final activity: Case study

Chloe is a play therapist and has just conducted her pilot study. Her research project aimed to explore the parent relationship with children who have selective mutism. Chloe has designed a semi-structured interview schedule to ask parents and their children about the challenges of daily life. However, she realised in the pilot phase that she was having difficulty engaging the children in the interview. She feels now that she should have spoken to stakeholders during the planning of the project to consider alternative methods for data collection.

A   **Activity   Planning for your project**

What advice would you give to Chloe at this stage to help her redesign her project to be more effective?

Having gained valuable experience and information from the pilot study, Chloe needs to start by re-focusing her research. Talking to stakeholders at this point would be valuable for Chloe in re-thinking how to approach her participants so as to give her a better chance of engaging the children. As quite a few changes are likely to be needed for the project to succeed, it is a great advantage to Chloe that she has realised this at such an early stage by having completed a pilot study. This means that time and resources and participant involvement have not been wasted by jumping straight into a full-scale but flawed research project.

Key messages

- The research question should be a timely area of enquiry which addresses a specific participant group in a particular setting.
- Proposals are important for convincing an audience of the value of your research.
- A research diary is a valuable tool in documenting and guiding the researcher in making important decisions.
- A pilot study is essential as a trial for the main project.

Further reading

Punch, K. (2000). *Developing effective research proposals.* London: Sage.

Sandelowski, M. & Barroso, J. (2003). Writing the proposal for a qualitative research methodology project. *Qualitative Health Research, 13*(6), 781–820.

White, P. (2009). *Developing research questions: A guide for social scientists.* Hampshire: Palgrave Macmillan.

CHAPTER 6

RECRUITMENT AND COMMUNICATION

Learning outcomes

- Differentiate between different types of sampling strategies.
- Recognise the different potential gatekeepers.
- Identify the challenges of recruiting children and families.
- Synthesise different communication strategies for gatekeepers and children.
- Recognise the importance of criminal record disclosure.

Introduction

We begin this chapter by discussing different types of sampling methods. Sampling and sample size are important considerations when beginning a project and these decisions will affect the rest of the process. Once you are clear about your sample population, it is likely that communication with gatekeepers will be a necessary starting point in recruitment. Many research projects recruit children through institutional settings and this may mean that you will need to navigate through several hierarchies of professionals before gaining access to families. This can be challenging and we provide clear guidance and examples to help you do this effectively.

Recruitment and communication

Recruiting children can be complex as the population of children (particularly those with health difficulties), is smaller than adult populations (Tishler, 2011). Recruitment and communication to engage children and families in research should be considered a process. There are many levels involved in recruitment and it is essential that you plan each phase. McCormick et al. (1999), state that there are four broad phases:

1. *Locating your sample:* There will be particular recruitment needs for different sites and places of recruitment and you need to identify these early on. Often institutions are multi-layered organisations and you are likely to have to go through a hierarchy of people before you can actually talk to children.
2. *Screening*: It is probable that your research question will require you to recruit a particular group of children for your research and you will need inclusion and exclusion criteria to help you screen your sample.
3. *Consent*: To recruit children to your research it is probable that you will need to gain informed consent from gatekeepers, parents and children. Children with mental health difficulties may have additional capacity issues which affect this process.
4. *Incentives*: You will need to make a decision regarding whether you offer incentives, financial or otherwise, to facilitate recruitment.

Additionally you need to think about other aspects of the recruitment process:

1. *Communication*: Your style of communication, modality of communication and language used will influence your recruitment success. Pay particular attention to the nature of the child's mental health difficulty as there may be intellectual impairments or social communication difficulties to consider.
2. *Professionalism*: It is necessary that you maintain a professional identity at all times.
3. *The motivation of families*: The reasons and motivations of families to participate in research will heavily influence whether they agree.

We now explore these issues in more depth and provide simple strategies for each element of recruitment and communication to apply to your own research.

Sampling

For your project you will need to recruit a sample of participants who are willing to take part. A sample is a group of participants that represents the broader population of individuals who meet the criteria of the research question.

> ### Example
>
> All children of a particular age group who have depression can be represented by a sample of children in that age group with the diagnosis.

The research question will guide your inclusion/exclusion criteria and may influence the kind of sampling procedure you choose to employ. In qualitative research it is argued that there are up to 24 different sampling techniques (Onwuegbuzie & Leech, 2007). With all qualitative sampling methods there are practical constraints, including time and resources, and therefore three of the most popular sampling strategies are listed below:

- A popular sampling strategy is convenience sampling. This is the least rigorous technique and involves the selection of the most accessible participants. However, while this is the least costly, it may result in poorer quality data (Marshall, 1996).
- The most common type of sampling strategy is purposeful sampling whereby the researcher makes an active selection of individuals with potential to provide rich information regarding the purpose of the research (Patton, 1990).
- An alternative approach is to use snowball sampling as a participant selection strategy. This technique involves building up a sample from existing participants' recommendations of possible additional people who may be approached (Blaxter et al., 2001). This technique can be especially useful when the population is difficult to identify through other means.

Sample sizes

Decisions about sample size are guided by the need to recruit sufficient numbers to address adequately the research question. In quantitative research your sample is likely to be quite large and is determined by a power calculation, but qualitative methods rely on smaller samples. There is no uniform agreement about exact sample sizes which has been universally agreed. Each methodological approach has its own quality criteria for sampling adequacy which should be adhered to. Recruiting too many participants can be problematic in that, first, an excessive volume of data can be unwieldy to effectively analyse, and second, it can be considered unethical to interrogate more participants than is necessary (Francis et al., 2010). As a general rule, in qualitative research small samples are acceptable and preferred (Tuckett, 2004) and in some cases a single case is sufficient.

The most commonly reported benchmark for deciding sample adequacy is the notion of saturation. A way of justifying sample sufficiency is by claiming either that thematic/data saturation has been achieved in the sampling process. Thematic saturation refers to a point in data collection when no new issues are emerging from the data (Francis et al., 2010) and this is an appropriate marker for many qualitative methodologies but not all (O'Reilly & Parker, 2013a).

Locating the sample

Once sampling decisions have been made your next challenge will be to identify potential locations and appropriate points of access to your chosen population, see Figure 6.1.

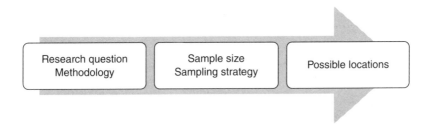

Figure 6.1   Access process

It is important that you plan ahead to think about the best way to access the population of children that you need. Although a specific location may seem an obvious place to recruit your sample it may not be the best place to conduct your research. For example, probation services may seem the obvious place to recruit young offenders, but security protocols may make this very difficult in practice. A second factor to consider is that perhaps access to a particular location for research purposes is relatively straightforward but it is not possible to recruit a representative sample. It may be necessary therefore to access children across several locations.

Gatekeepers

Gatekeepers are individuals who have some authority and may grant permission to access a particular group (Piercy & Hargate, 2004). An important aspect regarding whether you are able to recruit children with mental health difficulties to your study is the role of the relevant gatekeeper(s) and your relationships with them. In many settings adult gatekeepers are afforded responsibility for making decisions on behalf of children in their care (Heath et al., 2007) and part of this responsibility is to protect children and vulnerable families from intrusive research, or to ensure that situations are handled in a sensitive way (Heath et al., 2004).

It is likely that you will be dependent upon the goodwill of one or many gatekeepers for access to participants. In practice this is because access to children is typically dependent upon institutional gatekeepers and the legal position of children within society, although parents have a significant role and gatekeepers ultimately defer the final decision to them (Heath et al., 2004). However, institutional gatekeepers also play a significant role in the decision as to which children's parents you can contact (Scott et al., 2006).

> **!** Remember to be patient with gatekeepers. It is important to listen to their concerns and build rapport.

When planning your project it will be necessary to identify who the gatekeepers are. This will largely depend on the setting from which you plan to recruit (we discuss this in the next chapter in more detail). Each institution has its own policies, rules, regulations, relationships, structures and beliefs. It is important that you familiarise yourself with the procedures and structures of the institution you wish to recruit through if you are to successfully identify appropriate gatekeepers.

Example 1

If you are trying to recruit children in family therapy to a project then there will be several gatekeepers at the institutional level. This will include clinical managers and the practicing family therapists.

Example 2

If you are trying to recruit children who have suffered trauma or abuse then it is likely that you will need to have help from social services. This includes social services managers and practicing social workers.

> ## Example 3
>
> If you are trying to recruit children who have learning difficulties then you may choose to recruit through schools. This includes head teachers, special needs coordinators, teachers and possibly teaching assistants.

The number of gatekeepers you will need to liaise with will largely depend on the nature of your research, your research question and the characteristics of the sample you are trying to access. Sometimes there will be an overlap between institutions and this will make access more complex.

> ## Example
>
> If you wish to access children who are 'looked-after', such as children in foster care that are in therapy, you may need to communicate with clinical managers and therapists as well as social work managers and social workers.

Communicating with institutional representatives

To negotiate successfully with gatekeepers it is essential to build rapport with them (Emmel et al., 2007). It is likely that you are an outsider to the institution and will have to work hard to prove that you are professional and that your project is worthwhile. If you have existing relationships with gatekeepers this may help, but it is necessary to maintain a level of professionalism at all times being careful not to exploit those whom you know.

There are many different ways of communicating with institutional gatekeepers and you will need to make judgements about which is the most appropriate. We present some of these in Table 6.1.

Table 6.1   Forms of communication

	Individual	Group
Direct	Telephone Email Face-to-face Letter of invitation	Email Face-to-face Presentation
Indirect	Communication via acquaintances/colleagues	Information hand-outs Virtual notice board Website Leaflets and flyers

We suggest you use a combination of these approaches. For example, in seeking to recruit children from a school it may be advisable to make initial contact via a personal email or letter to the head teacher. This can be followed up with a telephone call to arrange an individual face-to-face meeting. You could take with you information in the form of hand-outs or flyers for the head teacher to distribute to relevant staff members and arrange attendance at the staff meeting to do a presentation.

Challenges of getting through the 'gate'

Gatekeepers can be a barrier to children having their voices heard rather than being a 'gate' through which their participation is enabled (Piercy & Hargate, 2004). This means that gatekeepers have the potential to silence and exclude children from research without actually consulting them (Alderson, 2004). It is important that you take steps to facilitate access and are aware of the potential challenges. We outline some of these challenges related to the institution in Table 6.2 and related to the research in Table 6.3, with potential solutions.

Table 6.2   Barriers to getting through the 'gate' related to the institution

Potential barrier	Possible solution
Time and pressure on the gatekeeper (Heath et al., 2007)	Remember gatekeepers are busy people so you need to be patient. Do not become a nuisance with constant demands on gatekeepers' time.
Institutional schedule (Freeman & Mathison, 2009)	Many institutions have particular time-frames, busier periods of the year, times when they are closed, specific times for lunch and so forth and it is necessary for you to adapt to these and not expect the institution to adapt to your needs.
Gatekeepers may be overprotective of children (Heath et al., 2004)	Gatekeepers are charged with protecting children's best interests so it is essential that you illustrate the ethical sensitivity of your research and the strategies and steps you are taking to protect them from potential harm.
There may be concerns about public scrutiny (Heath et al., 2007)	The gatekeeper may have concerns to protect the institution from exposure or negative findings. You will need to stress the elements of confidentiality, anonymity, and data protection. You should also make it clear that value judgements will not occur and that you will ensure consultation with them as the research unfolds.
Gatekeepers perceive the children to lack competence or to be too vulnerable (Heath et al., 2004)	This is a common conception amongst many adults, and institutional representatives. It is possible to try to convince them that you will take additional care that you have the skills to work with children in this category and that you will consult with them during the process, but ultimately they may deny access.

Table 6.3 Barriers to getting through the 'gate' related to research

Potential barrier	Potential solution
Gatekeepers may not understand what qualitative research is (Mander, 1992)	When communicating with gatekeepers you will need to carefully outline your project and the methods. Use a simple language and be prepared to answer any questions.
Your research project is not their primary concern (O'Reilly et al., 2013)	Your research project will be very important to you, but will not be their priority. It is helpful to indicate the potential benefits of your research and illustrate its importance. You will, however, need to give the gatekeeper time to respond to you.
The topic or the research methods may be deemed inappropriate (Heath et al., 2007)	Hopefully with careful planning, good supervision and consultation with stakeholder groups this will not happen. However, if they perceive it this way then you can show them your planning phases, provide them with details of stakeholder comments and provide evidence of reviews of your work. You can also answer their questions and provide reasons why the methods and topics are appropriate. You may want to use some research evidence to support this. Be careful not to try to 'blind them with science' though. Ultimately it is important that you listen to their concerns.

 Try not to be completely dependent upon a single institution as they may simply deny you access.

Ultimately you should respect the wishes of the gatekeeper. Remember they can facilitate or impede your research so be respectful and professional. Research illustrates that participants are more likely to cooperate and consent to participation if the gatekeepers have recommended it (Emmel et al., 2007) so it is essential to take the time to build good relationships at this level. Gatekeepers will draw upon their personal and professional experiences to inform their decisions as well as determining the perceived benefits of your research (Mander, 1992) so it is potentially helpful to try to gain some insight into their perceptions and feelings by asking them questions.

 If the children or families have poor relationships with the gatekeeper or do not trust them, they are then less likely to engage in your research project (Emmel et al., 2007).

A   **Activity   Identifying barriers**

Identify who the gatekeepers are likely to be in your research project. In your research diary make a list of all of the potential barriers you can think of for gaining access to your child participants. Alongside each barrier write down the ways in which you intend to overcome them.

In reality this means that there are four phases to recruiting participants and communicating with organisations effectively. These phases link closely with the phases outlined at the beginning of the chapter and were proposed by Munford and Sanders (2004):

1. *Contacting the organisation*: It is helpful to have a contact in the organisation that has regular contact with children and families.
2. *Inform the parents*: It is useful to arrange a meeting for all parents to attend to ask questions in groups. This can often be organised through the institution you are communicating with.
3. *Present the project to the children*: It is a good idea to meet with the children without the adults present and give them an opportunity to ask questions.
4. *Follow-up contact with parents and children and obtain consent*: This enables you to provide further information and offers another opportunity to ask more questions.

Recruiting children and families

Recruitment is essential if your research is to be successful and delays at this stage can cause significant delays to the project as a whole (McCormick et al., 1999). Recruiting children is especially challenging as their variable levels of competence and the nature of their difficulties can make communicating the value and risks of your project more complex. A fundamental aspect of recruiting children and families therefore will be your ability to communicate your research to them.

Communicating with parents

To gain access to your child sample you need to consider perhaps the most important gatekeeper, the parents. The law makes it clear that children under the age of 16 are not fully autonomous and this means that the parents may over-rule the child (Heath et al., 2004).

> ## Example
>
> The child may say that they do not want to participate in the research study but the parent may be enthusiastic. This may lead to the parent becoming coercive and trying to persuade the child to take part.

The parent may feel that your research is important and be keen for their child to make a contribution, or they may not like the child contradicting their authority (O'Reilly et al., 2013). If this situation arises then it is important that you respect the parent and handle the situation in a sensitive way to avoid compromising any parental authority but also to not push the child into your study.

> ## Example
>
> The child may be enthusiastic and want to join your study as many of their friends are taking part, but their parents may say no. This may be because the parent has fears regarding how the research will be used or simply because they do not have the time to facilitate it.

This can be very difficult, especially with older children. Although there are some circumstances where parental consent is not needed, generally the parents' decisions are final. Either way, wherever the potential conflict between parental and child views, parents do play a key role in consultations with children and it is up to you to do your best to communicate with them effectively. You need to provide accessible information about your project and illustrate any benefits/risks involved. Show the parents how long the child will be needed for, where exactly the research will take place and wherever possible negotiate any of the terms of the location, time-frame and use of refreshments, toys and so forth. You need the parents to help you to understand the child and his/her needs so it is important that you communicate effectively with this gatekeeper if you want your research to be a success.

Communicating with children

Communication is an intricate social process and one that is influenced by the characteristics of the individual, as well as the quality of the interaction (Pantell et al., 1982). Communication plays an important role in building relationships between professionals and children (McPherson, 2010) but often children's right to speak can be restricted and they must petition adults to enter a conversation (Pantell et al., 1982). When you are engaging children in your research it is imperative you pay attention to the communication strategies that you are using at every level. It is essential to communicate with children in a way that allows their voices to be heard and affords them a degree of empowerment within the process.

Typically we do not have a culture of listening to children and neither do we have a universally accepted set of procedures for engaging them in research (Munford & Sanders, 2004). It is your responsibility to learn about communication styles and consider what options are available to help children understand your project. It may be useful to have a range of tools at your disposal for communicating with children, including verbal/non-verbal techniques such as drawing and crafts (Thomas & O'Kane, 1998).

 Remember that children have the right to make their own decisions and it is important that you enhance this by outlining what is expected of them and what your research is about.

We can learn a lot about communicating with children who have mental health difficulties from the medical literature which seeks to advise health professionals on this issue. We present some practical tips in Table 6.4 to help you think about how to communicate with children, Table 6.5 for some specific guidance for communicating with children who have additional physical impairments and Table 6.6 for those who may struggle to understand.

Table 6.4   Communicating with children

Research situation	Communication strategy
Introducing yourself	You need to take particular care over your introductions. Let the child know how they can refer to you: first names are usually most appropriate. Make sure you know the name of the child in advance of meeting them and it may be useful to ask the child how they would like to be referred to (Willmott, 2010).
Child decision-making	The age and cognitive ability of the child may affect their ability to make decisions. Although older children tend to be more competent than younger children this will depend on many factors (McPherson, 2010). You should consider the child's cognitive functioning when asking them to make decisions and ask parents or professionals for additional guidance if needed.
Communication problems	By the nature of their mental health difficulty some of the children you engage will have communication difficulties. It is helpful if you talk to parents about any unique strategies they use to engage their children in conversations and look at the possibility of alternative communication methods such as voice output devices and multi-sensory references (Benjamin & MacKinlay, 2010).

Research situation	Communication strategy
Issues of language	When engaging with the child, be careful not to use jargon. Keep the language simple (Willmott, 2010). You may also need to use pictures or photographs to communicate, or use a computer (Benjamin & MacKinlay, 2010).
Written documentation	The research process will usually require you to present written information to children. Typically these are the ethics documents we talked about earlier in the book, such as information sheets and consent forms. It is useful if you provide this in a clear way to help you communicate with the child and you may want to use diagrams to facilitate understanding (Willmott, 2010).
Understanding the child	It is helpful if you have some prior knowledge of the child and family before you start as good preparation can help you to avoid problems (Benjamin & MacKinlay, 2010). Before you start talking to the child refresh your memory by going through any notes or advice the parents or professionals gave you and use this information to prepare the environment (Willmott, 2010).

Table 6.5 Communicating with children with physical impairments (Benjamin & MacKinlay, 2010)

Situation/impairment	Communication strategy
If the child you are researching has physical conditions	Some children in your sample may have physical impairments as well as mental health difficulties. You will need to do your best to offer them a comfortable environment, keep the research short so as not to tire them out and consider issues of access such as wheelchair ramps and disabled toilets.
If the child you are researching has a hearing impairment	You may need to think about having a communication aid, or an interpreter for sign-language. You will need a quiet room which is free from distractions.
If the child you are researching has a visual impairment	Children with visual impairments may miss non-verbal clues so it is important that you help them with this. The type of visual impairment will be important so you may want to think about the lighting in the room and keep auditory distractions to a minimum.

Table 6.6 Children who may have difficulty understanding/concentrating

Situation/impairment	Communication strategy
If the child has difficulty in understanding the research	It is important that you consider the level of understanding that the child has. The more complex the task you are asking of them the more assistance from you they are likely to need (McPherson, 2010).
If the child is anxious about the research	Sometimes children can be anxious about participating. It is important that you explain everything to them and offer them some reassurance. It is your responsibility to ensure they know what to expect (Willmott, 2010).
If the child you are researching has a learning disability	The child may therefore have difficulties with memory, concentration, attention or appropriate behaviour. Try to minimise any distractions and do not have too many toys available. Try to plan ahead and get advice about interaction from parents or teachers. Make some sensible decisions about what is developmentally appropriate (Benjamin & MacKinlay, 2010).

(Continued)

Table 6.6   *(Continued)*

Situation/impairment	Communication strategy
If the child you are researching has a condition such as autism or ADHD	Children who have these types of mental health difficulties are likely to have impaired social communication and may struggle to attend to the research for long periods. Try to make the child comfortable, choose a quiet environment and offer short breaks (Benjamin & MacKinlay, 2010). You may also want to consider more text-based communication such as Instant Messaging software, or email.

From this you should note that children are not a homogenous group and you need to consider the individual characteristics of the child, the nature of their mental health difficulties, any physical conditions they may have and their developmental age. It will be important to use specific communication techniques to facilitate understanding and enhance your recruitment and data-collection process. Remember that children's decisions cannot be made in a vacuum without the support from parents and professionals (McPherson, 2010).

Disclosure and Barring Service (DBS) formerly (CRB)

An important point for recruitment relates to your responsibilities when working with children. Many countries stipulate that a person must be police checked before having contact with children in a professional capacity. While internationally these checks differ there is much agreement that you need to be officially cleared before you can engage children. In the UK this is known as a Disclosure and Barring Service (DBS), which used to be known as a Criminal Records Bureau (CRB) check and depending on what you are doing you will require standard or enhanced disclosure. For children or vulnerable populations an enhanced check is usually required. The DBS check is a legal requirement put in place to safeguard children and you must allow time for this to be processed before you have direct contact with children in your research.

The DBS check has guidelines to ensure that conviction information is not misused and to ensure that ex-offenders are not treated unfairly and the Rehabilitation of Offenders Act (1974) allows criminal convictions to become 'spent' after a particular time of rehabilitation. Typically the more severe the penalty imposed on the individual, the longer the rehabilitation period. Once the conviction has been spent the individual no longer needs to reveal it.

 Some more serious offences such as most sexual offences cannot be spent and these types of offences are likely to affect whether you are able to work with or do research with children (O'Reilly et al., 2013).

You should be aware that when applying for your DBS check you will probably have to pay for this, unless your employer is willing to cover the cost. Additionally if it has been some time since you had one of these checks then it may be necessary for you to renew this for your new project.

Summary

In this chapter we have presented information related to the different sampling strategies and how to make decisions about sample size, inclusion/exclusion criteria and issues of location. We have provided some practical guidance on how to communicate effectively with gatekeepers; highlighted some of the potential barriers; and offered a case summary as an example. We moved on to describe the processes involved in recruiting children and families and communicating effectively with a wide range of children.

Key messages

- Qualitative sampling is different to quantitative and should be congruent with your methodological approach.
- The success or failure of your project may be determined by your relationships with the gatekeepers.
- Timely, appropriate and informative communication with parents and children is necessary.

Further reading

Benjamin, H. & MacKinlay, D. (2010). Communicating challenges: Overcoming disability. In S. Redsell & A. Hastings (eds), *Listening to children and young people in healthcare consultations* (pp. 151–168). Oxon: Radcliffe Publishing.

O'Reilly, M. & Parker, N. (2013a). 'Unsatisfactory Saturation': A critical exploration of the notion of saturated sample sizes in qualitative research. *Qualitative Research*, *13*(2), 190–197.

Willmott, A. (2010). Involving children: How to do it. In S. Redsell & A. Hastings (eds), *Listening to children and young people in healthcare consultations* (pp. 45–55). Oxon: Radcliffe Publishing.

CHAPTER 7

THE RESEARCH SETTING

Learning outcomes

- Distinguish different challenges associated with different research environments.
- Evaluate the issues in researching children in these environments.
- Assess the importance of the research setting.
- Appreciate the necessity of staying safe.

Introduction

In this chapter we explore the challenges specifically inherent in the research setting. We guide you through the issues you may face when engaging in child mental health research in particular environments. We start with clinical environments such as child mental health services and primary/secondary care settings and move onto other environments such as schools, community settings, homeless shelters and participants' own homes. As we address each setting we provide you with guidance for attending to the setting-specific issues and alert you to a number of features associated with that setting. The chapter concludes by considering your safety in the process of collecting data.

The issues

In any research setting there are four main considerations to take into account: choosing an appropriate setting, ethics, recruitment and data collection. Many of these concerns are pertinent regardless of the setting you choose and we have dealt with these earlier, in Chapters 4 and 6. There are, however, some challenges which are inherent to the specific research setting itself and we consider what these might be as this chapter unfolds.

Child mental health settings

Health professionals have an in-depth knowledge of the child's difficulties and are well placed to help you select suitable children for your research (Coyne, 2010). However, clinical professionals may view the children in their care as vulnerable and in need of their protection (Mander, 1992) and may see research participation as a 'burden' (Coyne, 2010).

Choosing an appropriate setting

There are many different child mental health settings which broadly fall into two types, inpatient and outpatient. Notably not all outpatient care occurs in the child mental health clinic, as it may happen in school or the child's home. Your choice between inpatient/outpatient will depend largely on what you want to find out. Typically researchers undertake research in inpatient care settings for more serious mental illnesses (Gans & Brindis, 1995) and outpatients for less serious cases. Part of your decision will relate to whether you are researching 'child mental health' as a broad category, whether you are focusing on one disorder or whether you are evaluating the effectiveness of an intervention/service.

Ethics in inpatient settings

It is not our intention to repeat material from Chapter 4 but remind you that general ethical issues are equally important. If you undertake research in clinical settings, particularly inpatient care, it is imperative you think about ethics in more detail. When considering the issues pertinent to conducting research in adult inpatient settings, Oeye et al. (2007) raise some important considerations, which are equally applicable to child inpatient settings:

- Inpatient psychiatric patients are considered especially vulnerable as they have impaired decision-making which can interfere with their ability to consent.
- It is necessary to cooperate fully with medical staff in judging capacity.
- There are doubts whether inpatient participants will benefit from participation.
- It can be challenging to observe individuals who have given consent in the inpatient wards without observing those who have not given consent.

 Remember that an institutionalised patient has been deprived of their autonomy (Radden, 2002) and this may be at odds with exercising autonomy in a research context.

Recruitment in inpatient settings

The recruitment issues you face may differ slightly depending on whether you are recruiting children from outpatient or inpatient settings. In addition to Chapter 6 you might need to think clearly about how you recruit from inpatient settings and the challenges that arise. Remember that institutionalised patients are often not free to leave the unit and have little control over who enters it (Oeye et al., 2007). This means that they have little say in whether you are allowed to access the communal lounges, dining areas, corridors, staff offices and other parts of the unit they may wish to visit. If you are given access by staff then you will need to be sensitive to this and consider how intrusive your presence is when you are visiting.

Data collection in inpatient settings

Our experiences of collecting data from young people in inpatient care have taught us that this is not a simple process. For example, qualitative research tends to rely on the recording of data (audio/video equipment), but this may be at odds with some inpatient settings where staff will not allow you to take equipment onto the wards. In practice you may have to do some additional negotiating to be able to take recording equipment in, take very clear field notes (which may not be as useful) or find an alternative form of data collection, for example asking participants to keep diaries and using those as data.

Primary and secondary care settings

There are many ways in which mental health is of interest in primary or secondary care and although we are bringing them together here, we are not suggesting that they are a homogenous group. There is great diversity across and within these settings but we broadly discuss them under the rubric of primary and secondary care to illustrate some of the specific issues of undertaking child mental health research in these areas.

Choosing an appropriate primary/secondary care setting

There are different types of primary and secondary care setting. Often these settings may focus on physical health but there are opportunities to explore mental health. Primary care is usually managed by GP practices, whereas secondary care bridges the gap between primary and inpatient settings and would cover a range of community settings where more serious mental health difficulties are treated.

Example – Primary Care

General practitioners are often actively involved in referring children suspected of having mental health difficulties to specialist services.

Example – Secondary Care

Paediatricians working in hospital environments may be actively involved in diagnosing conditions.

Example – Palliative Care

Those working in palliative care settings may be interested in the impact on a child's mental health when they have a terminal illness.

Ethical considerations in primary and secondary care settings

Again notwithstanding the ethical issues from Chapter 4, there are some inherent ethical challenges in collecting data in different clinical settings:

Time pressures:

- General practitioners may become stressed by interruptions to their workload (Pierce, 1998).
- Consent from hospital staff may need an on-going negotiation due to staff rotas and changes and different events unfolding on a daily basis (Wind, 2008).

Patient issues:

- Hospital/hospice professionals may resist your presence in the best interests of the patients (Wind, 2008).
- Terminally ill patients may believe that participating in the research has potential to help their condition and it will be important that you show this is not true (Terry et al., 2006).
- Palliative care research is ethically sensitive because of patients' vulnerability to having time taken up with research rather than spending their last days with their families (McWhinney et al., 1994).

Professional misconceptions:

- Some professionals may fear they will be judged as you scrutinise their work and may not understand why you are interested (Wind, 2008). It will be essential that you explain yourself.

Recruitment issues in primary and secondary care settings (physical health)

It is important that you communicate with professionals, parents and children effectively (see Chapter 6). Conducting research in general health settings differs from dedicated mental health clinics. Mental health may be important to these professionals, but physical illness is most likely to be at the top of their agenda. Recruiting from these settings can be difficult as professionals tend to be busy. It is important therefore that your recruitment strategy is as flexible as possible (Jordhoy et al., 1999). There are several things to be mindful of:

- Inform the whole practice/department so all members of staff, including administrative and security, are aware of what you are planning to do, how you are planning to do it and how the process might affect them.
- Inform all that there will be no financial rewards (unless you have funding) but that there will be small increases to their workload if they choose to help you recruit children (Pierce, 1998).
- When doing research in palliative care you need to be aware that complex symptoms, alongside physical and mental exhaustion may impede recruitment (McWhinney et al., 1994).

- When recruiting through gatekeepers, be mindful when they are likely to be most busy. It may be useful to leave your contact details and ask them to get in touch with you. It may be useful to write to them in the first instance so that you have a basis for your contact.
- Think about how you might recruit the children specifically. Research suggests that palliative care patients prefer to be approached about research by their caregiving doctor or nurse rather than a researcher directly (Terry et al., 2006) so it will be important that you have professionals helping you.
- Be aware that in palliative care research the patient may die before you have completed your recruitment (McWhinney et al., 1994) and therefore your recruitment process may take longer.

Data collection issues in primary and secondary care settings (physical health)

One concern when collecting data is the need to protect from infectious diseases. If you spend time in settings where infections are easily spread, then it is important you prepare for this. However, if there are additional issues in relation to the nature of the illness the child is suffering then make sure you communicate with the doctors regarding how to protect yourself. In terms of taking recording devices into potentially infectious environments, you will need to take precautions which minimise the risk of cross-infection to other patients. This can involve the need to prevent the device from touching any surfaces. You may also be required to wear gloves and/or a mask and disposable apron.

> **!** Remember if you have a virus then you could infect the child which may be serious if they already have a chronic condition. Regardless of how inconvenient to you or how minor your illness you should rearrange data collection when you are feeling better.

Schools

Conducting research in schools can be a useful way of obtaining data from children. Also, conducting your research in schools provides you with a way of accessing non-clinical and clinical populations, including those without mental health difficulties, those with mild mental health difficulties (but who have not sought help), those with mental health difficulties who are going through referral pathways and those receiving specialist interventions. This means that you can explore mental health very broadly, including mental well-being, stigma and bullying, as well as more specific aspects of mental health.

Choosing an appropriate school setting

In schools this is fairly straightforward as your choice will mostly reflect the age group of children you wish to engage. While internationally there are slightly different structures generally schools fall into four types:

1. *Preschool/nursery*: For young children in advance of going into a more formal school setting. The focus is still education but involves a lot more play activities and rest periods. Children tend to attend these for shorter hours.
2. *Primary/elementary*: For younger children of an educational age. The focus is on education and there is usually a standard curriculum.
3. *Secondary/junior-high/high*: For adolescents where the focus is on a standardised curriculum, making career choices and taking important exams.
4. *College/post –secondary education*: For older adolescents who wish to continue their education.

Ethics in schools

In schools there is an authoritative order between adults and children inherent in the nature of the educational format. Because of this there is a risk of coercion as children may view you as in a similarly powerful position to a teacher and might not feel they can refuse. Alternatively they may simply want to please you. You will need to ensure children can opt out or withdraw from your research. You will also have to take care over discipline. While working to empower children you may unintentionally contravene school policies or procedures and we recommend that you work closely with a staff member who can take responsibility for discipline. However, bear in mind that having a member of staff present is likely to affect the interactional dynamics and may even inhibit or distort participants' responses.

 Schools may be reluctant to engage in research on sensitive topics because of potential controversy (Gans & Brindis, 1995).

Recruitment issues in school settings

Recruiting children through schools is challenging and there are potential barriers. To help you understand this in the school context we provide you with practical tips for planning in Table 7.1 and for recruitment in Table 7.2.

Table 7.1   Planning recruitment through schools

Tip	Advice
Understand the structure of the school (Testa & Coleman, 2006).	Different types of schools have different structures, but even within one type of school there will be differences. Make sure you understand the administrative structure of the school you intend to recruit from, even before you make initial contact.
Get support from the parent/teacher association (Gans & Brindis, 1995).	Schools may question the legitimacy of your research so it is helpful to get support from outside of the school. For example the board of governors or the parent/teacher association.
Identify clear gatekeepers (Rice et al., 2007).	It is important to communicate with gatekeepers. In the school environment it is helpful if you can get a key teacher on board to support you in convincing other members of the school staff.
Conduct a pilot phase (Testa & Coleman, 2006).	If you have conducted a pilot phase of your research you will be able to inform the school how much time you need, how long the child will need to be out of the classroom for, how much commitment will be required from staff and children. This can be important in illustrating the minimal disruption to the school schedule.

Table 7.2   Recruiting through schools

Tip	Advice
Provide a clear summary of the research to teachers and head teachers (Rice et al, 2007).	Teachers need to be aware of how much they need to help you and what is involved for the children they care for. Provide a clear and succinct summary of the research and time-frame.
Provide an information pack (Testa & Coleman, 2006).	If the teachers are interested after reading your summary, provide them with more depth of information. You should give them an information pack which includes a second copy of the summary, a list of the research objectives, a summary of the potential benefits of the research, a copy of all consent forms, a review of the ethical guidelines, a copy of the questionnaire/interview schedule, and an information sheet. It is helpful to follow this up with a meeting for questions.
Collect consent at multiple levels (Rice et al., 2007).	You will need to collect consent from multiple levels including the head teacher, relevant teachers, parents and children. You may also need to collect consent from teaching assistants, educational psychologists or special needs coordinators depending on the focus of your research.

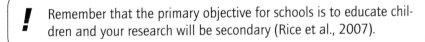

! Remember that the primary objective for schools is to educate children and your research will be secondary (Rice et al., 2007).

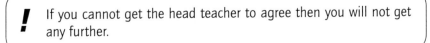

! If you cannot get the head teacher to agree then you will not get any further.

Data collection issues in school settings

The main issue here is when you collect your data. Schools have timetables and there are weeks in the year when children are away from school due to mandatory breaks. The other important issue in the school timetable is periods of exams. Teachers are not likely to want you to interrupt exam periods and use up revision time with your research.

 Remember that schools want to minimise the disruption to their schedules (Gans & Brindis, 1995).

You may also want to give thought to when you collect your data in terms of the time of day. While some children may be pleased to miss a lesson on a subject they dislike they will be less enthusiastic to miss out on an educational activity they find pleasurable. For some children missing sports may not be desired, for others a welcome opportunity. You may find it useful to consult with parents and children before you simply remove the child from a lesson they are enjoying. Equally if they are struggling with a particular subject it may be imperative that they do not miss those lessons. Some researchers choose to undertake their data collection during the child's break times or just after the school day. While this may be more appealing to parents and teachers you may find that the child is more uncooperative at these times. If data is collected during their break time (recess) they may miss out on being with their friends, if data is collected at the end of the school day then the children may be tired. Consultation with children, teachers and parents is important with all of these issues and try to work around their needs and not your own when scheduling in data collection times.

Community settings

In the literature there are many different terms for research in community settings including 'community-based research', 'community-involved research' and 'community-centred research' (Israel et al., 1998). There are, however, some key principles of this type of research as identified by Israel et al. (1998):

1. Views the community as a unit of identity. These communities of identity are centred on a defined geographic neighbourhood or a geographically dispersed sense of common identity.
2. Builds on strengths and resources within the community as it seeks to identify the resources and relationships that exist within communities.

3. Facilitates collaborative partnerships in all aspects of the research. The participants participate as equal members and share control over the phases of the research process.
4. Integrates knowledge and action for the mutual benefit of all partners.
5. Promotes a co-learning and empowering process that attends to social inequalities and which recognises that socially and economically marginalised communities may not have the power to name or define their own experiences.
6. Involves a cyclical and iterative process which includes partnership development and maintenance, problem definition, data collection and interpretation.
7. Addresses health from both positive and ecological perspectives.
8. Disseminates findings and knowledge gained to all parties.

Choosing an appropriate community setting

Again it is your research question that will help you determine which community setting to choose. There are many different ones which include:

- Youth clubs/centres.
- Skate parks.
- Sunday schools, churches or religious meetings.
- Activity/leisure centres.
- Drop-in centres.
- Children's groups such as Scouts/Girl-guides.
- Sports clubs (such as tennis, football clubs etc).
- Choir meetings.
- Dance classes.
- Gangs.

Each of these different community settings will have different concerns about your research in addition to the traditional ethical and practical concerns inherent in research generally. You will need to give some thought as to how the setting might influence the type of data you obtain and how or why that might matter in addressing your research question.

Ethics in community-based research

The main ethical challenge for community-based research relates to time as it takes considerable time to build relationships with community members/leaders before you are able to engage participants (Rawson et al., 2000). It can be problematic to determine who represents that particular community or to decide how that particular community is defined (Israel et al., 1998) and for some this may be more important than others. For example, in some ethnic or cultural groups, community leaders hold an authority which may help you to gain access to that community or may be ethically problematic if there is coercion. The culture of any community group (not just ethnic grouping) could be instrumental in your success and you need to understand it in advance of communicating with the children you wish to access.

Recruiting from community settings

Recruiting can be challenging as factors such as privacy, respect, religion, ethnicity, group culture and autonomy may affect your access. It is possible that conflicts may occur between members of a community (Israel et al., 1998) and therefore it may be difficult for you as an outsider to manage or understand it. Also, the community leader may not be an adult, for example if you are studying mental health in gang cultures the leader of the community may be under the age of 16 years which can make consent particularly challenging.

Collecting data in community settings

When collecting data in a community setting, you need to think about sampling. In community settings selective sampling is likely to be your starting point, as you have already selected a particular community or group to work with. If you are interested in the views and experiences of different members of the community, or from different angles, you may find that a mixed-methods design may be helpful. The temptation in community settings however, is to try to address too wide a topic, especially where community leaders may be taking an interest in your project and suggesting possible avenues of interest. Remember to stay focused on what question you are seeking to answer and the best methods to use to gather that data, without negating the views of the community themselves.

Homeless shelters and looked-after children

Although the focus of this section is on homeless and looked-after children, much of the information contained here also applies to other transient or mobile populations such as Traveller children and refugee/asylum-seeking children. Homeless children tend to display higher levels of mental health difficulties (Unger et al., 1997), which tends to be linked to previous experiences of recurrent mental health difficulties and their fragmented histories with mental health services (Taylor et al., 2006). Homeless children present with a range of different mental health conditions including anxiety, post-traumatic stress disorder and depression and present with risk-related behaviours such as self-harming and alcohol/substance abuse (O'Reilly, Taylor et al., 2009). Because of this research can be challenging but also rewarding and useful for developing interventions.

Choosing an appropriate homeless/looked-after setting

Deciding where to study homeless children will need careful planning, although choosing to study looked-after children may be more straightforward. With the assistance of social services it is possible to identify children who are looked-after by the State in children's homes or through foster care/adoptions. Each, however, presents different challenges. If you choose to do research with homeless children it can be very difficult to find them, although there are shelters and hostels directly set up for these populations.

Ethical issues in researching homeless/looked-after children

A major obstacle to undertaking research with homeless or looked-after children is ethics (Rew et al., 2000) which mostly relates to the problem of informed consent.

For homeless populations it can be difficult to obtain parental consent and trying to do so may actually endanger the young person (Rew et al., 2000). Children who are homeless are homeless for a reason and often it is because they do not want their parents to know where they are or because their parents do not care. This raises issues of how to gain consent from guardians and whether it is possible or morally viable. Nonetheless children under the age of 16 may not be able to fully consent for themselves, particularly if they have mental health difficulties.

For looked-after children a key issue is whether you need the consent of the birth parents in addition to the foster parents or State representatives (Bogolub & Thomas, 2005). Researchers seek parental consent for deciding what activities are in their child's best interests, but birth parents may not necessarily consider this (King & Churchill, 2000). Seeking consent from the child's birth parents can be time-consuming and may prevent a child who actively wants to participate in your research from doing so (Bogolub & Thomas, 2005).

> **!** If you choose not to seek the birth parents' consent it may be viewed as disrespectful (Bogolub & Thomas, 2005).

Recruiting homeless/looked-after children

Given the issues of consent it should be obvious that this is going to raise recruitment issues. Most notably with these populations is the number of gatekeepers that you may communicate with. It is probable that you will need to communicate with social services managers, social workers, foster carers, birth parents, children's homes representatives, hostel staff and the children themselves. Problematically these children are likely to be viewed as vulnerable and some of these gatekeepers may prevent children from participating even if they express a desire to do so (Heptinstall, 2000).

 You probably need the cooperation of social services to help you identify children to recruit and liaise with foster carers, homeless shelter staff, birth parents and so forth (Heptinstall, 2000).

Collecting data from homeless/looked-after children

An obvious difficulty in collecting data from these children is their transience. It is imperative that you give the children time to decide whether to participate, that you hold meetings so they can ask you questions and that you give them information in advance. Notably, however, as this process is unfolding some children in care homes or homeless shelters, hostels or other temporary accommodation will leave and others will come in. This transience can make it difficult for you to actually collect data from them.

Professional case example: Interview with Professor Vostanis

Professor Panos Vostanis (University of Leicester) has written extensively on child mental health in looked-after and homeless children. We asked him some questions about the challenges of doing research with homeless children and provide his responses below:

1 What do you think are the biggest ethical challenges of doing research with homeless children who have mental health difficulties?

When interviewing these children they seem to hope that you can help them get a house or that you might be able to help them therapeutically.

It's quite problematic that in their interviews they share abusive experiences but when the research is over there are no services to direct them to for help.

2 What were the hurdles you faced when recruiting these children to your research study?

The most difficult thing when trying to recruit young people who are homeless is the rapid turnover in any homeless shelter. These individuals move quickly and have changing circumstances which means that you cannot plan very easily.

3 What advice would you give to those who are new to doing research with homeless children who have mental health difficulties?

I would advise any researcher to be aware that they are going to need to work hard on this kind of project. It will be very important to get homeless shelter staff on board as they will be instrumental during recruitment and data collection. I would also advise the researcher to understand their systems and learn about what the shelter does. It is important in this kind of a project not to rely on others too much; allow plenty of time for recruitment and collection. This means that the researcher must make themselves available and be flexible and patient.

Some useful references

Meltzer, H., Vostanis, P., Bebbington, P. & Ford, T. (2012). Children who ran away from home: Risks for suicidal behaviour and substance abuse. *Journal of Adolescent Health, 51*, 415–421.

Taylor, H., Stuttaford, M. & Vostanis, P. (2006). A UK survey into how homeless shelters respond to the mental health needs of homeless young people. *Housing, Care and Support, 9*, 13–18.

Vostanis, P. & Cumella, S. (1999). *Homeless children: Problems and needs.* Jessica Kingsley Publishers.

There is more on his website: www2.le.ac.uk/departments/psychology/ppl/panosVostanis

Participants' own homes

Much data is collected in participants' own homes, particularly interview data, to alleviate placing additional demands on children and families (MacDonald, 2008). The family home is often recommended as a useful site for conducting research with children (Gollop, 2000). Because of this you may feel that it is appropriate to conduct your research in the child's home setting and this raises some particular issues.

Choosing an appropriate space within the home

The choice of room in which you collect your data is important for many reasons, not just technical considerations about recording quality and interruptions. The family home can be chaotic and may be more 'hostile' than you imagine it (Bushin, 2007). Some children feel more relaxed in their bedroom but take care not to assume that they have autonomy over this space (Punch, 2007).

 Be careful in terms of placing yourself in a situation where you are alone with a child as you may be vulnerable to suggestions/accusations of misconduct on your part.

Additionally, when talking about emotive subjects, it can be helpful to the child to do this in a more neutral environment so that these negative associations do not become connected to that place and the child still has a physical and psychological 'safe space' to return to after you have finished.

The negotiation of a private space can be a delicate matter (MacDonald, 2008) and you may not be able to insist that the television is switched off, the family pet is moved to another room or that seating arrangements conform to the research ideal (Bushin, 2007). You may also wish to consider your own personal boundaries and find out in advance, for example, if the family keeps pet snakes or spiders in the lounge. This has happened! All of these issues can make finding a suitable space in the family home difficult and in reality it is likely to require negotiation between allowing the child to choose where the research takes place and your own considerations. This should all preferably be negotiated prior to your arrival (Punch, 2007).

Ethics in the family home

Although the family home is often considered an ethically appropriate location as children tend to feel more comfortable there (Gollop, 2000) it does raise ethical issues. Mostly this relates to privacy and coercion. You are in a privileged position being invited into the family home so it is important that you are sensitive to the demands placed on the family, such as household demands, stress and parental occupations (MacDonald, 2008). While researching in the home does have the advantage that the child's peers are less likely to be aware of their participation (Bushin, 2007) there is a greater likelihood that your data collection process will be interrupted as other members of the household/visitors enter the room (MacDonald, 2008).

Recruitment issues when researching in the family home

The home environment is unpredictable and rapidly changing (Borbasi et al., 2002) and accessing children this way can be complex. To communicate with parents to set up data collection in their home, you will have to have the contact details of relevant families and usually this is achieved through formal or informal institutions. While you can advertise in public spaces, it is often easier to go through established institutions such as schools. If a particular sample of children is needed then you may need a good contact within the school to look through records and help you identify appropriate families to contact (Bushin, 2007).

Data collection issues when researching in the family home

By researching in the home it means that every situation will be different and this can be difficult to prepare for (Bushin, 2007). Bushin gives some tips for managing data collection:

- Understand the family's daily routines such as dinner times, bedtimes and so forth.
- Think about the time of day you see the child. Weekends may be more appropriate than evenings, or school holidays are good. Nonetheless be careful not to interfere with any plans they have.
- Be prepared to be flexible. Bushin noted that for three of the interviews she had planned when she arrived she found that the child was out with friends.
- You may have to be prepared to sit on the floor.
- You may have to stop the interview several times to accommodate interruptions.
- You will need good quality recording equipment as you may have little control over background noise.
- You will be less constrained by institutional schedules but remember that families have their own schedules.

Choosing your setting: A case study

Adrian is a clinical psychologist who wants to understand the impact on older children's mental health of not having their parents around. He is unsure at this stage whether he is interested in children who have been abandoned, who have run away from home, who are bereaved, or unaccompanied refugee children leaving their parents in the country of origin.

A **Activity   Deciding on a research setting**

Adrian comes to you for some advice. After considering the different difficulties related to different research settings, which group do you think Adrian should focus on?

Of course in reality Adrian should be guided by his research question, but practical realities of research settings may push him to refine his research question in relation to which group he can access.

Researcher safety

It is imperative to think about your safety during research. It is easy to focus on participants' well-being and forget about the risks you may take. Risk prevention in research is gradually being afforded more attention but it is still quite limited and the important area of risk management is still neglected (Parker & O'Reilly, 2013). Safety at work is a dual responsibility between you and your employer (Social Research Association, 2005) and your safety should be considered through a risk assessment (McCosker et al., 2001). Risk in qualitative research seems to present in two ways, physical and/or emotional, and we consider each of these in turn.

Physical safety

In research there have been occasional instances of physical violence, even death, and therefore safety should be addressed (Bloor et al., 2007). This can be complex as there is little literature on the physical threats that researchers face (Paterson et al., 1999) and researchers have historically tended to place less concern on physical than emotional risks (Sampson et al., 2008). Nonetheless preventing physical risk is important. If there is an obvious risk, such as the risk of infection, it is easy to focus on that and pay less attention to other physical risks. The risk is not necessarily higher for women than it is for men so be careful not to assume that gender makes a difference, although there is a higher risk of sexual assault for female researchers (Bloor et al., 2010). As protecting your physical safety is so important we provide you with some practical strategies in Table 7.3 when planning your project, some strategies in Table 7.4 in preparation for data collection and in Table 7.5 for collecting the data.

Table 7.3 Protecting physical safety when planning

Tip	Advice
Build safety into your funding bid.	It is useful to build in a budget for safety into your funding application which should include communication aids, risk assessments, insurance, extra fieldwork time, public transport and counselling (SRA, 2005).
Do a pilot study.	It is argued that a pilot study allows room to reflect on the dangers more carefully and implement stronger safety procedures (Sampson, 2004).
Get some training.	Researchers should receive training on how to handle threat, abuse or compromising situations (SRA, 2005).

Table 7.4 Protecting physical safety when preparing data collection

Tip	Advice
Research the neighbourhood before you visit.	Some neighbourhoods are known for their criminal activity and therefore it is important that you are aware of this and avoid where possible, or have plans in place if not (Paterson et al., 1999).
Consider any inherent dangers in the research setting in advance.	Remember for example that prisons/young offender's institutions can be dangerous places. Incarcerated individuals may become angry, hostile or resentful (Liebling, 1999). It is a good idea to do some research on the setting before you visit, ask staff for advice about any possible risks.
Change the venue.	If you feel at risk, or think that there may be issues then arrange to meet in a public space, but do not forget to maintain the privacy of the participants (Faulkner, 2004). If a public space is not possible due to the nature of your research and has to take place within a particular institution then make sure that you are aware of the institution's protocols and follow them.

Table 7.5 Protecting physical safety when collecting the data

Tip	Advice
Travel in pairs.	If resources allow it then collect data in pairs. The participants can be told that this is to help with the equipment, observe the method or assist with the data collection (SRA, 2005).
Use technology to help you.	Researchers should be equipped with alarm devices (Paterson et al., 1999).
Check in with someone.	It is a good idea for researchers to carry mobile (cell) phones to the interview, and report back to a supervisor as a method of enhancing researcher safety (Liamputtong, 2007).
Be careful what you reveal about yourself.	Do not give out any personal information; be cautious when leaving the participant to ensure you are not followed (Paterson et al., 1999).
Listen to your feelings.	Trust your instincts and follow your intuition. If you have a bad feeling about something then act on it and do so quickly (Paterson et al., 1999).

> ### *A* Activity   Plan for safety
>
> We recommend you read Parker and O'Reilly (2013). When you have gone through the main points make a list of all of the things that you think are important for protecting your own safety in your own research project. What physical risks might you face?
>
> - Parker, N. & O'Reilly, M. (2013). 'We are alone in the house': A case study addressing researcher safety and risk. *Qualitative Research in Psychology, doi:* 10.1080/14780887.2011.64726

Emotional safety

In reality physical risk is low and fortunately there are few reported cases of researchers coming to harm. A more prominent risk to your safety relates to your emotional well-being, particularly as in child mental health you are researching vulnerable groups and sensitive topics. Some topics are more sensitive than others (Johnson & Macleod-Clark, 2003) and it can be difficult to stay detached (Dickson-Swift et al., 2008), particularly as research on sensitive topics has potential to remind researchers of their own family's vulnerabilities (Coles & Mudlay, 2010).

You may find that your emotions range from mildly uncomfortable to personally disturbing up to traumatic, and some of these effects can last a long time after data collection is complete (Hubbard et al., 2001). Problematically this can lead to a risk of burnout as there is a cumulative response to traumatic material (Coles & Mudlay, 2010). This is an issue that you should take seriously and we provide practical strategies for managing emotional risk in Table 7.6.

The research literature does little to prepare the novice researcher for the reality of being out in the field (MacDonald, 2008) and therefore we have made some suggestions for how to deal with the risks you might face in our paper (Parker & O'Reilly, 2013) including:

- That there needs to be more attention paid to this area, with researcher safety being higher on researchers' agendas.
- Researchers should undertake some specialist training in staying safe and managing risk.
- The researcher should perform a transparent risk assessment.
- Researchers should debrief with their supervisors and should seek out support where they need it.

Table 7.6   Protecting emotional safety

Tip	Advice
Acknowledge your stress.	Data collection can be stressful and it is helpful to get some training on how to manage stress (Johnson & Macleod-Clark, 2003).
Take a break.	If a particularly upsetting/sensitive issue is the focus, then take breaks as this will be good for you and your participant (Hubbard et al., 2001).
Use a second researcher.	It can be useful to have a second interviewer who remains silent as this may ease the intensity of the one-to-one relationship (Brannen, 1998). Having someone else to discuss your emotions with can help with the activity of collecting data.
Make sure you have support.	More formal supervisory support to debrief can be a useful way of managing the emotional impact of the research (Brannen, 1998).
Use your diary.	You should be keeping a research diary which may be sufficient to record your thoughts and feelings.
Be prepared.	Certain topics may be more upsetting than others. Doing research with homeless children and hearing their stories of abuse can be emotionally challenging. Doing research with incarcerated individuals may be upsetting, or sitting with children who are dying, or have a dying parent, can be distressing. Make sure you have systems in place to look after your own emotional well-being.
Get some training.	Some specialist training in emotion management or counselling skills can be helpful, alongside good supervision (Johnson & Macleod-Clark (2003).

Overall we recommend that you consult the SRA (2005) guidelines which provide detailed guidance for researchers. Additionally there has been an inquiry which makes some important broad suggestions (Bloor et al., 2010):

- Researcher safety should be included in methods courses for students and therefore should be part of the pedagogical features of any course involving research.
- Major funding bodies should require researcher safety as an important feature for providing recognition to courses.
- Universities should provide training for supervisors and principal investigators and this should include researcher safety.
- All university departments should be subject to health and safety audits and there should be a section on researcher safety included.
- Funding bodies should require referees to comment on researcher safety issues.
- Ethics committees should have formal responsibility for oversight of provision for postgraduate student safety and there should be questions about safety on the application forms.

Summary

Although we have not exhausted all possible research settings for collecting child mental health data, we have considered many of them. We have considered which location within a setting might be appropriate, the ethical issues relevant, the recruitment challenges and the data collection difficulties related to that setting. While some issues are relevant to all settings and have already been discussed earlier in the book, each of these poses some unique issues for you to think about. We concluded this chapter with an often neglected consideration which is your own safety.

Key messages

- Choosing an appropriate research setting is essential to the research process.
- Different research settings pose different types of challenges for the researcher.
- It is necessary to plan for these challenges before undertaking data collection.
- It is imperative to stay safe in the field, undertake a risk assessment and take care of your physical and emotional safety.

Further reading

Bloor, M., Fincham, B. & Sampson, H. (2010). Unprepared for the worst: Risks of harm for qualitative researchers. *Methodological Innovations*, *5*(1), 45–55.

Gans, J. & Brindis, C. (1995). Choice of research setting in understanding adolescent health problems. *Journal of Adolescent Health*, *17*, 306–313.

Parker, N. & O'Reilly, M. (2013) 'We are alone in the house': A case study addressing researcher safety and risk. *Qualitative Research in Psychology*, doi: 10.1080/14780887.2011.64726

PART THREE
DATA COLLECTION

CHAPTER 8

QUESTIONNAIRES, OBSERVATIONS AND ETHNOGRAPHY

Learning outcomes

- Describe the process of designing questionnaires, observations and ethnography.
- Differentiate between different types of data collection.
- Judge the appropriate information needed in the data collection design.
- Compare the benefits and limitations of each method of data collection.

Introduction

There are many different approaches to collecting data from children and in this chapter we focus on three common types: questionnaires, observations and ethnography. Each of these modalities has important benefits with some associated limitations and challenges. We provide you with practical guidance to choose which data collection methods are most appropriate for your research question and to help you with the design of your study. We consider ways to design questions in order to elicit useful and important information from the children about their mental health experiences and to make necessary decisions regarding the number of questions required and the type of language to utilise.

Questionnaires

At some point you have probably been asked to fill in a questionnaire. The purpose of a questionnaire is to ask participants questions in a structured and systematic way. They tend to be quantitative in nature, although can be qualitative or have some qualitative questions built in. There are several different ways to administer questionnaires to children and we present the most common in Table 8.1.

Table 8.1   Administering questionnaires to children

Self-administered (Those filled in by the participants)	Researcher-administered (Responses recorded by the researcher)
Post	Face-to-face
Internet	Telephone
	Administered by a gatekeeper

 Activity   Experience of questionnaires

Think back to the last questionnaire you received and in your research diary write down the reasons why you did/did not fill it in.

It is likely that your personal motivations for filling in questionnaires include the nature of the topic, the purpose of the research, the length of the questionnaire, the layout and format. These are also influencing reasons whether professionals, parents or children might agree to complete your questionnaire. It is important that you think about these issues when you start to construct your design.

Developing your questions

An important thing to remember is to keep your questionnaire child-friendly, especially for qualitative questions. The first thing to decide is the nature of your questionnaire as you may want to engage in one main type of questioning or combine them.

- Closed (yes/no) questions.
- Open (what, where, how, why, when) questions.
- Rating scales.
- Likert scales.

It is important that you give some serious consideration to the differences between these different types of questions before you begin. The examples below may help you to decide which format is most appropriate for your research design.

Example closed question: Do you feel happy when you are with your friends?

Example open question: How did you feel when you were admitted into hospital?

Example rating scale: On a scale of 1–5 (1 being low, 5 being high) how anxious do you feel when you arrive at school?

Example Likert scale: Please circle answer to the statement 'I feel less anxious now I am on medication' – Strongly Agree – Agree – Neutral – Disagree – Strongly Disagree.

Questionnaires often use closed questions and these are quantitative in design. Children are required to choose from pre-existing responses such as yes/no or true/false. This type of question can be good for children as it requires them to provide a definitive answer. Open questions tend to be qualitative and are designed to elicit more detailed responses from children. Open questions may be a useful addition to your questionnaire as they allow for more free responses, but be aware that some children may struggle with this depending on their literacy ability and how much help is available to them. Also, questions need to be worded clearly and carefully, in a way appropriate to the child's age.

Children can be particularly susceptible to giving what they think are the 'right' answers. Think about how you might consider the impact of social desirability in responses.

Likert scales and rating scales elicit different types of responses as they provide children with a scale or set of statements requiring them to determine the extent to which they agree/disagree, or how they rate something on a scale. You will need to pay attention to the breadth of the scale and the options you provide children with. Having a 'don't know' or 'neutral' option may lead to many children simply ticking this box rather than really thinking about their answer. We provide you with some practical tips for designing questionnaires in Table 8.2, with a specific focus on questions in Table 8.3.

Table 8.2   Tips for designing your questionnaire

Tip	Description
Make sure you ask only one question at a time (DeLeeuw et al., 2004).	When designing your questionnaire remember that one single question at a time should be asked so as not to confuse the children. Keep each question relatively short and clear.
Make sure your questionnaire is focused on the topic and related to the aims of the research (O'Reilly et al., 2013).	It is important that the responses children give you to the questions on your questionnaire actually provide you with the knowledge you are seeking. To ensure this you need to make sure that the questionnaire is designed in a way which is focused on the main topic under investigation and is relevant to the aims of your research.
Be careful not to make assumptions about your participants.	Just because the participants are children you need to be careful not to make assumptions about their interests, feelings or mental health difficulties.
Proof read your questionnaire before sending it out.	Make sure that you check the spelling/grammar of your questionnaire before you give it out.

Table 8.3   Tips for designing your questions

Tip	Description
Do not use leading questions (O'Reilly et al., 2013).	Make sure that your questions are as neutral as possible.
Use unambiguous and straightforward language (Bell, 2007).	Remember that children may take questions literally and therefore it is important to remove any ambiguity. Make sure your questions are written in a child-accessible language. It can be useful to ask some children you know to critically appraise the questions before you finalise them.
Include questions which contradict earlier ones (O'Reilly et al., 2013).	It is important that you check that the child is not just ticking random boxes. To do this you can include questions which address the same issue with a different construction so that to tick the same box would contradict the answer to the original question.

> **!** Remember that much child mental health research is sensitive in nature and therefore you will need to design your questions with this in mind.

A Activity   **What is wrong with these questions?**

Have a look at the three questions below and decide why they are examples of very poor questions for a child mental health questionnaire:

1 Please circle the answer which best represents what you think is the aetiology of your condition? A) Predisposing genetic factors – B) Biological manifestation of symptoms – C) Environment and societal impact.
2 How do you feel when the bedroom lights are turned out, why do you feel like this and what physical feelings do you have at this point? Try to explain why you feel scared of the dark.
3 We think children with anorexia nervosa simply don't enjoy eating food, do you feel this way? Please circle your answer. Yes – No

---

Hopefully you noticed that question one is ambiguous. It contains complex terminology which children are unlikely to understand, such as 'aetiology', 'predisposing' and 'manifestation'. This is likely to cause confusion, meaning that your participant will not understand the question. Additionally the question uses the concept of 'condition' when it would be better to actually put the condition name into the question, such as ADHD, depression or whatever it is you are researching.

Question two is long, contains too many elements and the child is unlikely to be able to answer it. It asks the child to articulate how they feel about the dark, to provide an explanation for why they feel this way and to explain any physical symptoms which may simultaneously occur. Essentially this question also makes assumptions as it presupposes that the child is afraid of the dark rather than openly asking how the child feels.

The third question is also poorly constructed and hopefully you recognised that this question is leading, containing potentially inaccurate information. This question simply reflects the researcher's own personal view and is not grounded in any of the evidence on eating disorders. Because of the way the question is phrased it encourages the child to answer in agreement.

Designing your questionnaire

Once you have designed your questions it is important to go back to the literature to help you refine them. It is useful to test your questions on children you know of a similar developmental and chronological age as the participants you plan to use. Deciding on the exact number of questions to include in your design can be difficult and will depend on the topic and the question you are addressing. The length of your questionnaire will rest ultimately on the age and abilities of the children who will be responding to it. It is important that you keep the questionnaire as short as you can. Research tells us that longer questionnaires generally have lower response rates than shorter ones (Roszkowski & Bean, 1990) so we advise that you try to keep your questionnaire to a maximum of two pages.

 It is always best to keep questionnaires designed for children as short as possible.

The next step is to start thinking about the broader issues of questionnaire design. You need to think about the layout of the pages, the length of time it may take the children to respond and the need to pilot it. There are three important things that you need to remember:

1. *Have an introduction sheet*: Do not make the assumption that the children automatically know what to do. Your questionnaire should contain a simple introduction giving them instructions about what they need to do, how they should do it and roughly how long it may take them to do so (Holoday & Turner-Henson, 1989). You may find it useful to provide an illustrative example as part of this to explain it better to children.
2. *Have a bright and clear layout which is appealing*: Remember that these questionnaires are designed for children so try to make the layout appealing to them. Depending on the format in which you are presenting the questionnaire you may want to include animation features, pictures or diagrams which help the child to answer the questions, but also make the questionnaire look more interesting.
3. *Pilot the questionnaire*: It is essential that you pilot your questionnaire before you administer it to your participant group. You will then need to consult your pilot participants to see how they found the exercise, what problems they encountered and whether any questions need clarification or re-designing. You can use the feedback to revise your questionnaire.

Some children may have difficulty reading the questions and may need someone to read the questions out loud to them. This may, however, introduce some bias that you need to be aware of.

Benefits and limitations of using questionnaires with children

When developing your questionnaire it is important you consider the broader benefits and limitations of the design. Be clear about why you think that a questionnaire is the most suitable approach with which to address your research question and do what you can to counter any limitations inherent in this method. We provide some of the key benefits and limitations in Table 8.4.

Table 8.4   Benefits and limitations of questionnaires with children

Benefits	Limitations
Because you can make the questionnaire relatively short, the child is less likely to become bored when filling in their responses.	The nature of some mental health conditions mean that concentration is poor and therefore the child may require someone to sit with them while they fill in their responses.
Well-designed questionnaires have potential to provide you with a significant amount of useful information.	If the questionnaire is poorly designed you will end up with a lot of information which fails to address your research objectives.
If the questionnaire is systematically organised then it is unlikely that the child will fail to answer any of the questions.	If the questionnaire is less well designed the child may fail to answer some questions and this may mean that you cannot include that questionnaire in your sample.
Questionnaires tend to be a cost-effective method of data collection.	There is often a requirement that questionnaires should be validated and this is time consuming and potentially expensive.
Closed questions enable the child to provide a quick response and allow for speedy data entry for analysis.	The child may struggle to answer some of the questions although hopefully the use of a pilot will have eliminated this possibility.
Questionnaires can be used with children from most different age groups, social and ethnic backgrounds, and with both boys and girls.	Closed questions do not provide space for the child to explain their answer and some children may be reluctant to be so 'black and white' about an issue.
	The child may not have the educational level or cognitive/linguistic abilities to fill in the questionnaire. You may find a face-to-face method works better.
	Children may give socially desirable answers or simply circle the same response for all questions (more common with rating/Likert scales). Including contradictory questions can help with this.

Observations

Observations are one method of data collection which form a wide range of research activities and can be quantitatively or qualitatively performed. Observations can help us to improve our understanding of an individual, a relationship, a social group or culture (Greig et al., 2007). There are four main types of observation which are commonly used with child participants (Greig et al., 2007) and we outline these in Table 8.5.

Table 8.5   Four types of observation

Type	Description
Controlled/structured	Controlled observations are those which are to some extent manipulated by you. Some refer to this as a structured observation (Robson, 2011), where you take a more detached position from the observation and usually quantify behaviour through predetermined coding schemes (quantitative).
Naturalistic	This is a form of observation whereby you observe the child or children in a more natural environment without intruding on the space. The clinical setting can be considered a more natural environment if it is part of their usual routine and not imposed for your research study. Using a naturalistic observation can give a 'real world' edge to your study and can be useful for children with mental health difficulties.
Participant	This form of observation is one where you become a participant in the setting. You become part of the context that you are studying and communicate with the children you are observing.
Non-participant	This is where you simply observe from the sidelines or where you observe discreetly without telling the children they are being watched. This does of course carry ethical concerns and may need to be well justified.

These four different types of observation can be combined:

Example

You may decide to undertake a participant naturalistic observation where you join the children in their natural setting and become part of that world. So you may observe children in a school classroom to see how their mental health needs are being met.

Example

You may decide to undertake a non-participant controlled observation where you sit discreetly and watch children. This approach is common with many training courses that require infant or nursery observations.

For a nursery observation for example, you may be interested particularly in recording a number of themes such as interactions with other children, responsiveness to adult carers or choice of play resources. These can be observed discreetly whilst sitting unobtrusively in a corner of the room.

There are different ways of noting down the children's behaviour and meeting the objectives of your research. This will heavily depend on the nature of your project and the purpose of it. You may choose to actively audio- or video-record the observation so that you have a good record of what happened, although obtaining ethical consent may be more difficult. Alternatively you may choose to rely on your notes or checklist. For some observations the presence of a recording device may be too obtrusive.

 Try to keep any recording equipment as unobtrusive as possible and place devices discreetly in the environment (Greig et al., 2007).

Whatever format you decide is most appropriate you will need to take notes during the observation. According to Willig (2001) there are three different types of notes that you can take during your observation and these are outlined in Table 8.6.

It can be difficult to make notes during the observation, particularly if you are observing many children. It helps if you can write short-hand or develop your own system of symbols so that you can write more quickly. You may find it helpful to type up the notes or copy them to your research diary when the observation is complete so that you can be aided by your recent memory.

Table 8.6 Types of researcher notes (Willig, 2001)

Type	Description
Substantive	These types of notes need to feature as much detail as you can capture including concrete descriptions of the setting, people or events.
Methodological	These notes will reflect your role in the research and your relationship with the participants. You can also note down any problems that you encounter during the observation.
Analytical	You may want to note down any analytical ideas that you have as you watch the children. Record any emergent patterns that you see or any themes that you think are emerging as this will help facilitate the beginning of data analysis.

> ### *A*   Activity   Practice making notes
>
> It is worth practicing this activity to see what it is like before you do your project. Set up a ten-minute observation with children you know. See what happens and how well you do. Make your own list of the challenges you may personally face when making notes.

Personal case example: Making notes

The first author undertook a series of observations for her undergraduate degree (rather a long time ago!) of children in the classroom. There were ten children in each observation so this meant a lot of information to capture. Lots of notes were scribbled down and several pages were produced. A few days later she found that she could not read all of her own writing and some information was simply lost. It can be quite easy to lose the coherence of your notes when writing quickly and your writing may become untidy. This is why it is very important to rewrite them or type them up as soon as you can, even if you have neat handwriting.

Making notes during an observation is not straightforward. Children may question what you are writing and may wish to contribute (Knupfer, 1996). You may decide this is acceptable and give the children some paper to write down their thoughts, but this may distract from the main activity you are observing or the children may take over your note-taking completely leaving you with a limited set of notes. You might also want to consider having more than one observer present if you are observing a group of children to reduce the likelihood of some behaviour being missed.

>   While having more than one observer can improve reliability there is the risk that disagreements may occur between observers.

Ethnography

Ethnography is a qualitative design which aims to explore cultural phenomena. Ethnography tends to rely on observation methods and typically ethnographers use participant observation techniques. This is a feature which distinguishes it from other methods (Hammersley, 1985). The term ethnography means to write about people and the way they understand and make sense of their experiences. It is through ethnographic work with children that we are able to explain their everyday social lives (James, 2001). The main purpose of ethnography is to gain an understanding about a specific group, such as children with mental health difficulties. Ethnography is a particularly useful method to use with child participants and has been helpful in recognising children as individuals competent in their own social worlds (James, 2001). Typically when you start your ethnography you will be a stranger to the children and their families and you will need to put in effort to build rapport and encourage the children to be open (Christensen, 2004). Ethnography takes place over a reasonable length of time and to do ethnography effectively you will need to be highly engaged in the process.

> ❗ Getting accepted into children's worlds can be challenging as there are some obvious differences between adults and children in terms of cognitive and communicative maturity, power and physical size (Eder & Corsaro, 1999).

If you choose to conduct an ethnographic study then you do need to be mindful of the practical and methodological requirements to do this effectively. Remember ethnography often requires long-term fieldwork over a period of time so that you can immerse yourself into the children's world (Eder & Corsaro, 1999), so you need to be sure that the project time-frame allows this. There are four main advantages to ethnographic work with children and it can be a particularly useful method for studying mental health:

1. Some children who have mental health difficulties have limited competence or speech and therefore it may be appropriate to observe them rather than use more verbally dependent methods.
2. Ethnography is a useful method for allowing more marginalised groups, such as children with mental health difficulties, to voice their perspectives and have those voices heard. This method advocates a children's rights perspective and promotes the view that children are competent to illuminate their own worlds.
3. Because ethnography tends to favour naturalistic observations you are able to observe the child in their natural environment and as an active participant you can spend lots of time with the child to truly understand their perspective.
4. This method allows you to immerse yourself in the field of study and really learn about children's world and yield important knowledge about child mental health experiences, perspectives and attitudes.

Ethnography can be a very appealing method as it allows for a more holistic picture to emerge and is a flexible method of data collection. You may be interested in spending time with children with mental health difficulties to help you build up a picture of their worlds. However, ethnographers are highly skilled, well-trained researchers, so do be careful not to underestimate the work involved in this kind of research. There are some limitations of this method that you ought to consider before you develop your research plan:

1. As we noted, to do ethnography effectively it is very time-consuming.
2. Ethnographers are highly skilled and you will need training which will require time and resources.
3. Gaining access to some social settings may be difficult, particularly because of the high level of involvement you will need to have. It can be quite difficult to convince people to allow you to spend so much time in their environment.
4. Children are important gatekeepers in ethnographic work as they allow you access to their social worlds so significant effective communication will be needed in the negotiation process (Warming, 2011).

Summary

This chapter has introduced you to three common forms of data collection in research. Questionnaires, observations and ethnography can be useful methods to collect data from children about their mental health. Questionnaires are typically quantitative and we have provided practical guidance regarding how to design one and how to use this method effectively with children. In our discussion of observations we differentiated different types of observation and placed a particular focus on ethnography.

Key messages

- Your questionnaire should be child-friendly, not too long and contain sensible questions.
- It is important that you take clear and detailed notes during your observation of children.
- Ethnography can allow you access to children's worlds and is linked to your view of children and childhood.

Further reading

Bell, A. (2007). Designing and testing questionnaires for children. *Journal of Research in Nursing*, *12*(5), 461–469.

Hammersley, M. (1985). Ethnography: What it is and what it offers. In S. Hegarty, & P. Evans (eds), *Research and evaluation methods in special education* (pp. 152–163). Philadelphia: NFER-Nelson.

O'Reilly, M., Ronzoni, P. & Dogra, N. (2013). *Research with children: Theory and practice*. London: Sage.

CHAPTER 9

INTERVIEWS AND FOCUS GROUPS

Learning outcomes

- Distinguish between different types of interviews.
- Carry out interviews/focus groups with children.
- Recognise the changes necessary for children of different age groups.
- Critically assess the potential value of participatory methods.
- Discuss the limitations of interviewing/focus groups.

Introduction

In this chapter we introduce the techniques of interviewing and focus groups. We integrate our discussions of the two methods as although focus groups are not just a 'group interview', there are many similarities. We open the chapter by introducing the different types of interviewing, which provides a platform for your decision-making. This theme continues as we provide some practical strategies for interviews and focus groups with children. One of the contentious issues regarding research with children is the use of participatory methods. Whilst some authors automatically include additional techniques to help engage children, particularly those with mental health difficulties, others take issue with this automatic inclusion. In this chapter we guide you through this debate, while introducing you to some of the more commonly used participatory methods.

Introducing interviews

Interviewing is a popular technique (Kvale & Brinkman, 2009) and is the most common method of data collection for qualitative research in healthcare settings (Britten, 2000). Research interviewing is different from clinical interviewing. Clinical interviews vary depending on the context and purpose. Medical interviews for example, are often quite structured and largely designed to establish facts. In contrast the research interview usually tends to be more interpretive with a goal of shared understanding (Borbasi et al., 2002).

There are different types of research interview and we introduce you to the three main types in Table 9.1. The boundaries between these are, however, more complex than is often considered and the terminologies are understood differently by researchers representing different qualitative approaches. Nonetheless they remain a helpful heuristic to guide researchers in broad terms.

Structured interviews are associated with quantitative research. These are based on the idea that factual information can be directly accessed through asking specific questions. If you choose to carry out a quantitative structured interview then you will be required to gather data using scripted questions which are administered in precisely the same way for all participants (Roulston, 2006). While quantitative structured interviews may be useful in some contexts, the premise that it is possible to access information directly has been challenged by some (Wooffitt & Widdicombe, 2006).

Table 9.1 Types of interview

Interview type	Description
Structured interview	The structured interview is associated with quantitative research and involves rigidly going through a series of questions.
Semi-structured interview	The semi-structured interview is a qualitative method whereby the researcher has an agenda and a loose schedule of questions, but there is flexibility.
The unstructured interview	A qualitative method involving some questions but the interview is unstructured and more like a conversation around a theme.

Semi-structured and unstructured interviews are qualitative and there are some similarities. Both types of interviews favour open questions (Wilkinson et al., 2004) and it is through the interview that the researcher attempts to understand the world from the participant's point of view (Kvale, 2006). A semi-structured interview is one whereby you have a general schedule of questions but there is some flexibility regarding how many of those questions you ask and in what order you ask them. In this way the semi-structured interview is organised around this set of pre-determined open questions with supplementary follow-up questions designed to elicit more detail. An unstructured interview is similar but the participant is afforded significant control over the direction and content and although the interviewer plays an active role in guiding it the participant leads it (Corbin & Morse, 2003). An unstructured interview will resemble a conversation, although this reference to dialogue is misleading as conversations suggest mutual interests but this is not the case in the interview (Kvale, 2006).

Example

In a new field of research where the evidence-base is limited a researcher may choose to conduct unstructured interviews as a way of exploring the issue in a general way. In an area with a significant volume of literature, however, researchers may draw upon this evidence to formulate more directive questions, while still giving the participants scope to express themselves freely.

 Even if you are familiar with clinical interviewing it is advisable to get some research interview training before you start your research.

Introducing focus groups

Focus groups generally require a small group of children brought together to discuss a particular issue. Focus groups are similar to group interviews but there are some differences. A focus group allows the discussion and development of a topic with some direction from the moderator, whereas in a group interview the moderator has much more control, following the schedule of questions more closely. Nonetheless in a focus group it is your responsibility to guide the conversation and follow the research agenda. You should set the tone and manage the flow of the group discussion and decide which topics to pursue and which to abandon (Hoppe et al., 1995).

Interviews with children

Up until the mid-1990s qualitative interviewing of children and families was avoided, mostly because it was believed that children lacked the social competence to recall credible accounts of their experiences (see Morrow & Richards, 1996) or because researchers felt uncomfortable about lacking the skills needed to interview children (see Harden et al., 2000). This was further complicated by the complexity of accessing children through the many layers of gatekeepers (Mauthner, 1997).

However, despite a slow start, interviews with children are now quite commonplace. The goal of interviewing is to invite children to give their own perspectives and by choosing to interview them you issue this invitation (Danby et al., 2011). If you interview children you will need to gather background information on your participants so that you can take into account their age, linguistic and cognitive ability, developmental stage and attention span (Wilson & Powell, 2001). Before you plan your interview consider your role in it:

1. *Question your own assumptions:* You should not rely on your own assumptions during the interview. Instead you should check that you have understood correctly the meaning the participant was trying to convey (Britten, 2000). With children this is especially important as their maturity, language and communication skills are developing.
2. *Consider your clinical status:* If you are clinically trained some of those clinical interviewing skills can be transferable but you do need to monitor your technique (Britten, 2000). Ask others to critically appraise your pilot interviews.

There are many practical issues that you need to consider at the planning stage of your interview and we provide you with some practical advice in Table 9.2.

It is important to prepare children for the experience and build up rapport. Rapport is usually established by taking time before the interview to get to know them, but with children this is more time-consuming. One meeting with a child is not likely to be sufficient as children tend to be wary of unknown adults (Irwin & Johnson, 2005). Remember that while rapport is essential, you need to be cautious about suggesting your relationship is a 'friendship', particularly if your participants are vulnerable (Borbasi et al., 2002). Although Borbasi and her colleagues were considering vulnerable adults, their observations are also important in relation to children, particularly in terms of how they may react to your disappearance after completion (e.g. children with autism). It would also be wise to have a fairly good understanding of the mental health difficulty that you are seeking to research further in order to take into account any specific factors relating to building rapport or maintaining

Table 9.2 Tips for planning

Tip	Description
Decide interview type.	You need to decide whether the structured, semi-structured or unstructured interview type is most appropriate (Kvale & Brinkman, 2009).
Plan carefully.	Plan the interview carefully and obtain demographic information from parents/schools regarding their age, competence, likes/dislikes and anything else that may be relevant to your study (O'Reilly et al., 2013).
Decide how many children you need.	Make decisions regarding the appropriateness of your sample size (Kvale & Brinkman, 2009). Bear in mind that the objective of qualitative research is to sample the range of views, and as such there is no one method for 'selecting' qualitative research participants (Gaskell, 2000).
Consider length of your interview.	Consider how long your interview will last, bearing in mind that they typically last approximately 45 minutes (Peters, 2010). With children however, depending on their age and concentration, you may need to make that shorter or you may choose to have a break halfway through.
Consider your interview environment.	In advance of the interview you will need to prepare the setting, which is particularly important for a child. Pay attention to the way the furniture is arranged so that you and the child are on an equal level, such as on cushions on the floor, and avoid sitting behind a desk (Cameron, 2005). Remove any clutter or toys so that the children do not get distracted by them, but with young children you may wish to have some in a box in case you need them to engage the child in communication (Wilson & Powell, 2001).

engagement with your sample population. This can make your job more difficult but there are some ways to overcome it depending upon time, resources and cooperation from others:

- Arrange to meet the child in advance of the interview at least once. You could visit the child in school/home and in the presence of parents/teachers to build up a relationship prior to the interview.
- Allow longer for the interview so that you have time before you start to get to know the child. Perhaps spend some time playing with the child, asking about his/her hobbies/toys/favourite food or television characters.
- Ask parents to prepare the child for the interview. You could even give them a photograph of you and ask them to give the child lots of verbal information about what to expect. We had a comment from one child which was '*I thought you would be fatter and wearing pink*', said with some disappointment.
- Be mindful that children are not likely to be experienced at being asked for their views or participating in interviews and they may have some anxiety about what is involved (Cameron, 2005).
- You could have a conversation with the child over email or telephone to explain what will happen.
- Remember that some methods require multiple interviews or multiple forms of data collection so you will be spending quite a lot of time with the child and family. Some children may miss you when you have gone.

> Remember that the goal of interviewing children is to allow them to provide you with their own personal perspectives and it is important you provide them space to do so (Danby et al., 2011).

Undertaking interviews with children may feel daunting if you have not done this before. Children communicate differently to adults and if you are new to this you may feel some anxiety yourself, which can make it more difficult to put the child at ease. Be prepared and think about the interview in a practical way. In Table 9.3 we outline some practical strategies to help you start the actual interview and in Table 9.4 some practical hints to help you develop your skills.

Table 9.3 Tips for getting started

Tip	Description
Prepare your participant.	Before the interview begins talk to the child about the process and manage their expectations. Inform them of the purpose of the interview, draw their attention to any written information and clarify ethics (Corbin & Morse, 2003).
Reassure your participant.	At the beginning reassure your participants by reminding them that there are no right or wrong answers (Wilkinson et al., 2004). You may find that children need this more so than adults as they are used to educational environments where specific 'right' answers to questions are expected.
Relax your participant.	Before you start spend some time engaging in small talk to help them relax (Corbin & Morse, 2003). You may have to change or adapt your interviewing technique for each individual child to make sure that the interview suits their needs (O'Reilly et al., 2013).

Table 9.4 Tips for conducting your qualitative interview with children

Tip	Description
Give the children a degree of control over the interview.	It is helpful to adopt strategies that enable the participants to control their degree of exposure and maintain valuable narratives about their lives. In sensitive topics particularly, questions should be prefaced tentatively in an effort to open choices for participants (Sinding & Aronson, 2003).
Think about your questions.	It is important to use open questions and avoid leading the participant to a particular type of answer. Try not to ask 'why' questions as participants often have difficulty pinpointing their personal motives and avoid asking abstract questions (Wilkinson et al., 2004). With young children however, the space for their contribution can make them feel uncomfortable and thus it is better to start with simple closed short answer questions to help them to relax into the interview (Irwin & Johnson, 2005).
Think about the order of your questions.	When dealing with sensitive topics it is important not to launch straight into sensitive areas. Try to start broadly with less emotional areas and move into the more sensitive questions later (Corbin & Morse, 2003).
Deal with distress appropriately.	When interviewing individuals about sensitive topics there is a risk they may become upset. Make sure you are prepared for this, have tissues available, be empathic and non-judgemental and remind them they can stop the recording and that they can withdraw if they wish (Corbin & Morse, 2003).

Focus groups with children

The focus group is an ideal forum for enabling vulnerable groups to express their views openly in a supportive group setting (Powell et al., 1996). It therefore allows children to express a range of opinions and experiences with space for challenges by other members. Focus groups with children allow you access to children's own language and cultures, encouraging elaboration of issues and concerns (Singh & Keenan, 2010). You do need to be careful when using focus groups with children as they may become uncomfortable talking about sensitive topics. Be aware of the possible cues of this discomfort but be mindful that comments and giggles may illustrate that, despite embarrassment, the children are willing to continue talking (Hoppe et al., 1995).

There are many things that you can do to ensure that your focus group goes smoothly. In Table 9.5 we provide some practical advice when preparing your focus group, in Table 9.6 we provide you with tips for starting one and in Table 9.7 are tips for conducting your focus group. Additionally many of the practical tips for interviewing also apply to focus groups.

Table 9.5 Tips for preparing focus groups with children

Tip	Description
Arrange seating to promote equality (Morgan et al., 2002).	It can be helpful to sit on the same level as them to ensure a sense of equality. This does not mean that you lose your identity as an adult as you will need to facilitate communication and step in if conflict arises.
The background and expertise of the researcher is important (Fraser & Fraser, 2001).	If you are new to focus groups it can be helpful to have a focus group moderator with some expertise and experience working with you.
Think about how you dress (Rauktis et al., 1998)	You need to consider what you wear to the focus group and how you present yourself. A formal outfit may give an impression of authority which may expand the power differential, but something too casual may give the wrong impression too.
Consider the environment and the furniture (Rauktis et al., 1998).	For those with mental health difficulties you will need to think about their comfort and the arrangement of the furniture. Make sure they have comfortable chairs and consider whether a table is obtrusive.
Think about the location of your focus group (Rauktis et al., 1998).	The location of your focus group is important. You may think that it is convenient to use a room within the mental health service as children are familiar with the setting, but they may find it more difficult to provide any negative comments about the service if they fear service providers are listening.

Considering the child's chronological age

The way in which you carry out your research, at least partially, will depend on the chronological age of the child and the nature of their mental health difficulty. While the practical tips we have given you so far will be useful for

Table 9.6   Tips for starting focus groups with children

Tip	Description
Give the children and yourself a name tag (Hoppe et al., 1995).	It can help to relax children, particularly if they are unknown to each other, if they wear name tags. It is important that you also wear one and identify yourself as a member of that group. It could be fun to have an 'art' activity before the focus group commences where the children design their own name tags as this can break the ice.
Make sure you introduce the focus group properly and the members (O'Reilly et al., 2013).	Introduce yourself to the children and remind them why you are there. Make sure all children introduce themselves to the group, and outline the goals of the research in a child-centred way.
Create a list of rules (O'Reilly et al., 2013).	Sit with the children at the beginning and allow them to draw up a list of rules they think they should follow during group discussions. You may need to guide them to be respectful of one another but the activity can be insightful.
Differentiate the focus group from group therapy (Rauktis et al., 1998).	Some children with mental health difficulties may have been engaged in group assessments or group-based interventions so it is important that they understand that the focus group is not a therapeutic intervention.
Start with general issues and move to specific (Hoppe et al., 1995).	Hoppe et al. (1995) noted that if the topic is sensitive it is especially important that you start your focus group with less sensitive issues and gradually move to the more sensitive topic questions. This allows the children to get used to talking to each other and allows you to become familiar with them.

Table 9.7   Practical tips for conducting focus groups with children

Tip	Description
It can be useful to provide refreshments (Morgan et al., 2002).	Children may find it difficult to concentrate for the length of time and therefore it is a good idea to have breaks roughly every 20–30 minutes.
Create a dialogue and be collaborative (Farquhar & Das, 1998).	Creating a dialogue with the children is fundamental if you are going to be inclusive and collaborative. This can encourage conversation and reduce power differences.
Be careful not to allow some children to dominate the group (O'Reilly et al., 2013).	The focus group setting may be inhibiting for some children and they may be less inclined to voice their opinions. Other children may enjoy contributing and dominate the conversation. As the moderator, work to elicit contributions from quieter members and carefully stop any single child from dominating the conversation.
Allow children to ask questions at the end (Hoppe et al., 1995).	It is useful if you allow enough time at the end of the focus group for children to ask you questions about the group and about the research more generally.

your project you do need to consider the individual capabilities of the child. Broadly we consider three age groups: neonate to four years old, school-age of five to eleven years and adolescents, twelve to eighteen years. We of course recognise that within these ranges there is great diversity and the different types of problems increase this variability significantly. Nonetheless, it is worth thinking about some of the general differences between the age groups so that you may then individually tailor your interviews/groups to suit.

When conversing with children there is usually reliance on language and very young children may be difficult to engage. This is something you need to think about when considering the appropriateness of interviewing or focus groups. Most very young children, for example, are likely to have limited competence to engage and it is likely to be difficult to create reliable meaning from their talk, because with issues such as grammar, semantics and syntax there is a risk of misunderstanding between you and the child (Cameron, 2005). If you choose to interview children this young then you will need to keep it short, you may want to consider having the parents present during the interview to make a contribution.

If you make the decision to interview (or use focus groups with) young children (aged five to eleven years) then you need to ensure that your communication techniques reflect those children's interests, experiences and values (Christensen, 2004). Remember that this age group have a tendency to give answers that they believe you want to hear so you will need to phrase your questions carefully and check their answers back with them. Avoid using leading questions, particularly those that encourage yes/no responses. As we mentioned in Table 9.4, you may find it useful to give these children some control over the interview and encourage them to tell you stories (O'Reilly et al., 2013), but there are also some additional practical issues to think about:

- This age group will be at a particular developmental stage regarding language (which may be delayed as a consequence of their mental health difficulty) and therefore this is something that you need to familiarise yourself with. We recommend that you spend some time with children of this age group by volunteering with a youth group or school.
- If you have limited experience working with children then you may find it useful to seek some advice from teachers, parents, or others and gather specific information about the children you are planning to interview. Find out more information about their preferred communication styles.
- You may want to provide some refreshments for these children. Be careful however, to check with the parents that they are happy for their children to be given these products and be aware of allergies. Also, if breaks are planned in you need to make sure that these are not too long or distracting so that you can easily re-engage children's attention when you restart the discussion.

> **!** If the child has language/communication problems then you may need to think about how much you rely on verbal techniques, favouring instead text-based interviews or the use of photographs/pictures (O'Reilly et al., 2013).

If you decide to interview (or use focus groups with) older children (aged twelve to eighteen) then you need to alter your style and questions. Researching this group is different from younger children as they are likely to have a greater capacity and understanding. This in itself means that you will have to hold the attention of your participants and keep the interview interesting. Things to remember about this age group:

- There are greater demands on their time in terms of school work, exam stress and peer relationships.
- They are going through physical and emotional changes associated with puberty/adolescence.
- Because they are older they may have a better understanding of the informed consent process but they are still minors and safeguarding remains an important issue.
- This age group may also have anxiety about participating for fear of negative recourse from peers or feeling foolish. You will need to help them feel more relaxed and reassure them that there are no wrong answers.
- You will need to think about the language you use and the tone of your communication. Be careful not to patronise them or pretend to be part of their group.

Developing a schedule

If you are going to use interviews or focus groups, then you will need to develop an engaging schedule. This topic guide is an essential part of the process and needs to be designed in a way which captures your aims and objectives (Gaskell, 2000). Again it is important to think practically about how you develop this schedule and we provide you with guidance in Table 9.8.

Table 9.8   Tips for developing an interview/group schedule

Tip	Description
Use the literature.	The questions asked should be guided by the literature. By doing this you should have a sense of the themes to be investigated and a conceptual and theoretical knowledge of the area (Kvale & Brinkman, 2009).
Ask for help.	Your schedule should be guided by others in your team, or other professionals. Have discussions with experienced colleagues and foster a more creative thinking style when developing the questions (Gaskell, 2000).
Think about the format.	The schedule should not be too long as you should follow the answers given by the participants and respond accordingly. Roughly the schedule should only be one page focused around broad headings which reflect the research agenda (Gaskell, 2000).
Do not be rigid.	Do not use the schedule as a rigid guide, it is a guide only and simply assists you in the questioning process (Wilson & Powell, 2001).

Remember that the schedule is only a guide and is NOT a script to be followed meticulously (Gaskell, 2000).

 A   **Activity   Try it yourself**

Try to devise three broad areas of interest for your own research and try writing at least two clear questions for each area. Show them to a colleague who is experienced and ask for feedback.

Deciding whether to have the parents present

A central issue you will need to address is whether to speak to the children alone or ask parents to be present. Sometimes you may not have much choice if either party specifically request it. Sometimes the child may be alone, the parent may be present (but quiet), or they may actively contribute to the answers (Irwin & Johnson, 2005).

Whether parents are present or not will depend mostly on the child. Some children are shy and find sitting with strangers uncomfortable, so allowing the parent to stay in the room can help to put them at ease which helps you to build rapport. Although you may have some concerns that the parents may interrupt or interfere potentially compromising the integrity of the interview/group, this is rarely the case. Parents tend not to lead children, particularly in an interview context, and if they do make contributions then this tends to scaffold the child's responses adding richness to the child's stories and giving a sense of completeness that you may not have otherwise achieved (Irwin & Johnson, 2005). If the child has particular mental health difficulties then the parents' presence can actually help. If the child has behavioural problems then the parent will be able to take responsibility for any aggressive outbursts or may be able to facilitate the child's attention. If the child has learning delay then the parent may be able to help you rephrase questions so that the child is able to answer them for you.

Alternatively however, older children may be less likely to disclose information if their parents are present (Mauthner, 1997). Some parents find it very difficult to let go and want to hear everything that the young person has to say and if this is contrary to the wishes of the child then you will need to take some control. One technique for facilitating this is to reassure the parents that you have a duty to disclose information if any safeguarding issues arise.

The use of participatory methods

The use of participatory methods has become popular, with a range of activities being drawn upon to engage children in research in a more meaningful way (Coad & Lewis, 2004). Traditionally participatory methods were used to engage disadvantaged adult populations, but with an increased use in child research they can be especially helpful for doing research with children who have mental health difficulties (Liegghio et al., 2010). The literature proposes several arguments for why participatory methods can facilitate research with children:

- Participatory methods provide an epistemological advantage as they produce better types of knowledge than other methods (Gallagher, 2008).
- Participatory methods are more ethically acceptable than other methods as it helps to provide children with a 'voice' (Gallagher, 2008).
- Using participatory methods can allow the child to shape the agenda and give them some control over the research (Thomas & O'Kane, 1998).
- Using participatory methods can provide a mechanism for children to talk about more complex and abstract issues (Thomas & O'Kane, 1998).
- Participatory methods allow a more meaningful participation with vulnerable populations as they allow them to participate as collaborators with the power to make and influence research decisions (Liegghio et al., 2010).
- Participatory methods have the potential to empower children as they take control of the activity (Waller & Bitou, 2011).

There are many different types of participatory methods, including: drawing, photographs, poetry, dance, glitter pens, emoticons, vignettes, story-telling, drama, games, video, mapping and song. If you choose to employ some additional participatory activities in your interviews/groups then we do recommend that you read additional texts on this subject. We do, however, provide you with an overview of four of the most common techniques.

Arts and crafts   Drawings

The use of arts and crafts is one that children are familiar with. This can be an especially helpful aid if you are seeking to engage very young children or those with limited verbal ability. The act of drawing can help to take the focus away from you as a researcher and provide a more child-centred way of sharing the child's experiences (Driessnack, 2006). Asking the child to draw pictures, or use other artistic techniques such as glitter pens, wool or pasta shapes to create art can help to encourage trust and motivation, ultimately improving communication (Horstman et al., 2008). However, be careful about imposing your own interpretation onto drawings and where possible ask the child to explain their work.

! It may be helpful to leave the child for a short time, allowing them to concentrate on their drawing. You should stay in the room and answer any questions, but try not to interrupt the child's flow (Horstman et al., 2008).

Photographs

With changes in technology there has been an increased use of photography in child research. Asking children to take photographs can help you appreciate their personal experiences as they facilitate the elicitation of information. Photography as a form of visual story-telling can promote participation of children as they get excited by the use of the cameras (Drew et al., 2010). By giving disposable cameras to those who find it difficult to express themselves, the method can promote social inclusion and emphasise the capacity of vulnerable participants rather than their incapacity, taking the focus away from deficit (Aldridge, 2007). You need to be careful, however, how you explain this in your ethics proposal, and consider what boundaries would be appropriate to put on this method and what you will do with the photographs.

! Some children may find it difficult to know what to photograph and may find it challenging to represent their illness or experiences visually (Drew et al., 2010).

Vignettes

Vignettes can be used as a tool to elicit children's understandings of their own experiences by making reference to a third party. Vignettes may be presented as text, pictures, on the computer, by video, or through the internet. In the vignette the researcher presents a story and the participant is asked to respond to that presented situation by imagining what they think the third party should do, how that third party might feel, or how the third party might have done things differently. Remember that children do not always feel confident when talking

(Continued)

(Continued)

about themselves and using a vignette allows them some space to explore their experiences and draw parallels with the individual represented in the vignette (Barter & Renold, 2000). If you are doing research with young children then you need to make sure that your vignette is not too complex and can be easily followed (Barter & Renold, 2000). Choose vignettes with children of a similar age and perhaps background or culture if this is relevant to the study. Alternatively you can use cartoon characters or animals in vignettes.

! Make sure that your vignette contains sufficient context for the participants to have an understanding of the situation but is vague enough to allow them to provide the additional factors which influence their judgements (Barter & Renold, 2000).

Communication aids   Toys and pictures

You may not want to overload your research with participatory methods and therefore you may choose something simpler, like toys or pictures representing emotions. Communication aids such as picture prompts can be especially useful for sensitive topics, with faces showing different emotions being a helpful technique for eliciting the child's feelings (Hill, 1997). For example:

Figure 9.1   Communication aids: Faces

! Make sure that you do not use abstract pictures with the children; the emotion should be clearly interpretable. Also note that some children due to their mental health condition may have perceptual difficulties in 'reading' emotions in others.

While it may seem obvious to use some additional activities within the interview/group to encourage children to talk to you and foster a partnership style of communicating, it is important to note that the use of participatory methods is contentious. They are not always needed as some children will be happy to sit and chat to you about their problems without the need for additional encouragement. Participatory methods grew out of shifts in thinking about children and childhood, a movement which sought to reposition children as agents with rights, as competent social actors (Gallacher & Gallagher, 2008). We considered this in Chapter 5 where we talked about how your views of children affect and shape the way you do research.

Your view on children's position within society will also affect your decisions about participatory methods. One of the arguments about their usage rests on the assumption that children need to be empowered by adults, with the idea that the use of additional activities allows children to exercise their agency (Gallacher & Gallagher, 2008). You need to exercise caution, however, as in isolation the activity does not empower children; it is your discussion with the children that creates opportunities for them to create meaning in relation to their experiences and it is this shared engagement that promotes empowerment (Waller & Bitou, 2011). Furthermore by emphasising participation it may actually reduce possibilities in the research encounter, as their usage necessitates a predefined activity and this may actually constrain possibilities for them to act (Gallacher & Gallagher, 2008). Ultimately any additional participatory methods must remain flexible to suit a range of developmental capabilities (Drew et al., 2010) and you must use your common sense.

Problems with interviews

As we mentioned, interviewing is a popular method to collect information from children but there are several issues you should consider when deciding its appropriateness. It is important to challenge the popularity of interviewing and its priority as first choice, as its effectiveness should not be taken for granted (Potter & Hepburn, 2005). There are several problems with interviewing children and we list these below:

- The interview context may feel quite formal and frightening to some children, particularly younger age groups, and so you will need to make sure that you help the child relax.
- You need to think about the nature of the mental health difficulties that your participants are experiencing. Interviews may not be the most suitable mode of inquiry for children who find articulating their views verbally difficult.
- It is easy to slip into using more adult-type language in the interview as you progress through it. Remember that you must maintain child-friendly language to keep the child engaged throughout the process.

- There is a risk that the child may not say much during the interview and therefore you need to be prepared for this.
- Your data may not get to the child's actual experiences and instead it may be unduly biased by the interview process. In other words the child may provide you with socially desirable answers as they may feel anxious in your presence.

The value of interviewing has been questioned by some and it can be challenging for novice researchers to understand how to use interviews in ways that are congruent with the theoretical and epistemological assumptions which underpin the design (Roulston, 2010).

Case study

Charlotte is a trainee child psychiatrist interested in how mental health professionals communicate with their child patients. She decides to use semi-structured interviews with a range of professionals from child mental health services, social services and charitable organisations. She decides also to interview child service users about their experiences of being communicated with.

> ## *A*   Activity   The usefulness of interviews
>
> We recommend that you read the paper by Potter and Hepburn (2005) and review this chapter so far and then attempt to decide whether interviews are the most appropriate way of learning about communication and child engagement.
>   What might be an alternative data collection strategy for Charlotte?

While interviewing may be useful for Charlotte to use there are several issues she needs to think about. There are a number of advantages to using interviews with both the professionals and the children:

- Interviewing provides Charlotte with a flexible method for data collection which can be adapted for both professionals and children. A semi-structured schedule allows her to ask different types of questions to different groups and change the wording to suit the participants. Charlotte also has the opportunity to use some participatory methods for children who are less verbal or have communication difficulties.
- Interviews are a useful way for Charlotte to engage the child and the professional in dialogue about their experiences of communication. Charlotte will be able to pursue any interesting ideas that either participant talks about.

- Interviews can provide Charlotte with depth of information and she can use additional probing answers to encourage the participants to expand further.
- Interviews are a useful method to explore sensitive issues such as mental health communication.

If you have read the paper by Potter and Hepburn and reviewed our checklist in this chapter you may decide that interviewing is not the most appropriate method. Problematically, professionals and children are reporting on how they communicated in a previous context and this relies on their memory and interpretation. Often people think they perform better in that context than they actually do which will affect the way it is reported. It may be simply that Charlotte only gets a reflection of the interview itself rather than really looking at the communicative practices.

Problems with focus groups

While focus groups are useful for gaining multiple viewpoints it is important to consider how you will deal with the inherent disadvantages:

- Studying groups brings with it issues such as conformity, children's relationship, dominant/passive members and group dynamics. As the facilitator you need to be aware of this and encourage quieter children to contribute, deal with silences, bullying or conflict and balance your authority against empowering children and giving them some equal status.
- Sensitive topics require you to handle them sensitively. You need to ensure that the conversation does not become distressing for some children and you need to take care to supress any gossip that may occur once the focus group has ended (O'Reilly et al., 2013). Remember, however, that what is sensitive to one child may not feel as sensitive to another (Farquhar & Das, 1998).
- Some individuals will not reveal information in a group context, because of the fear that this information may be revealed outside of the group (Kitzinger, 1994).
- There is a risk that children will adopt themes offered by other children rather than offer up their own opinions or experiences (Lewis, 1992).
- It can be quite challenging to coordinate a mutually convenient time and place to get the children together. This will depend on your recruitment strategy and where the children are geographically placed. You will be dependent upon parents bringing their child to the venue and you may need to think about the expense associated with this.
- You need to be aware that transcribing focus groups can be more time-consuming as there are multiple parties speaking and an increased likelihood if overlapping speech or interruptions.

Personal case example: Focus groups with children

The second author was involved in a project which used focus groups with 10–14-year-old boys discussing issues related to emotional health education in schools. The boys' school was selected because there had been a suicide and staff and parents felt that education on mental health would be a valuable addition to the curriculum. The focus groups formed part of a pilot project whereby a series of mental health issues had been covered in weekly tutorial lessons, including depression, self-harm and suicide. Three groups were run with seven boys in each group and the groups were also video-recorded. The aim of the focus group discussions was to elicit information on how the boys had found the teaching materials, what they had learned, how it had influenced their thinking and views about the stigma of mental health difficulties and whether they felt that the information could be delivered differently.

A   **Activity   Choosing your method**

From looking at the case example above what do you think the benefits of using this method were for a) exploring mental health and b) doing research with this age group?
   What (if any) advantages might there have been from doing a questionnaire design with some open questions instead?

The focus group was chosen as the most appropriate data collection method as the topics covered were sensitive and being part of a group gave the boys the option of choosing to respond to a particular question or not. It was also chosen as preferential over individual interviews as the boys could hear one another's perspectives and thus it was hoped that this would facilitate a more open attitude to discussing these topics with less social stigma. With boys of this age it is usually the case that talking about such sensitive topics as this would typically be quite difficult and boys are usually less likely than girls to discuss emotional or mental health difficulties with peers for fear of bullying.

Summary

This chapter has introduced you to some of the important practical and theoretical considerations you need to make if you decide to employ interviewing or focus groups as your data collection technique. Undertaking interviews and focus groups with children is different from with adults and we have provided you with some practical strategies to encourage child participation and engagement. Additionally we have debated the value of participatory methods with vulnerable groups such as children with mental health difficulties, giving you some practical advice on how best to use such additional activities.

Key messages

- Broadly there are three different types of interview technique: structured, semi-structured and unstructured.
- Different age groups and developmental capabilities will require different techniques and styles to elicit information.
- Interviews and focus groups are useful for eliciting children's illness experiences but there are disadvantages which ought to be considered.
- Participatory methods can help to foster a partnership with children, empower them and give them a greater degree of control over the research agenda.

Further reading

Britten, N. (2000). Qualitative interviews in health care research. In C. Pope & N. Mays (eds). *Qualitative research in health care* (pp. 11–19). London: BMJ Books.

Farquhar, C. & Das, R. (1998). Are focus groups suitable for sensitive topics? In R. Barbour & J. Kitzinger (eds), *Developing focus group research: Politics, theory and practice*. Thousand Oaks, CA: Sage.

Kvale, S. & Brinkman, S. (2009). *Interviewing: Learning the craft of qualitative research interviewing* (Second edition). London: Sage.

Wilkinson, S. Joffe, H. & Yardley, L. (2004). Qualitative data collection: Interviews and focus groups. In D. Marks & L. Yardley (eds), *Research methods for clinical and health psychology* (pp. 38–55). London: Sage.

CHAPTER 10

NATURALLY OCCURRING DATA

Learning outcomes

- Distinguish between researcher-generated and naturally occurring data sets.
- Identify the different ways in which naturally occurring data can be collected from clinical settings.
- Debate the challenges of collecting and analysing naturally occurring data.
- Recognise the value of using documents in research with or about children.
- Evaluate the usefulness of collecting diaries as data in child mental health research.

Introduction

We open this chapter by making an important differentiation between two categories of data collection. In the literature it is argued that there are data 'generated' by the researcher or data which are naturally occurring. We start by providing an explanation of the differences between researcher-generated and naturally occurring data and provide an overview of debates relating to the categorisation of different types of data source and their utility for different kinds of qualitative analysis. The relevance of this debate is made transparent in our discussion of the ways in which naturally occurring data sets can be utilised in child mental health research. A clear and practical discussion is provided regarding how naturally occurring data can be collected from clinical settings and we provide some personal research examples. The chapter concludes with a more specific focus on one of the types of naturally occurring data by exploring the potential use of documents in child mental health research.

Differentiating researcher-generated from naturally occurring data

Often researchers do not consider whether the type of data they are collecting is researcher-generated or naturally occurring. It is common for researchers to opt for interviews or focus groups due to their popularity and familiarity. It is important, however, to have an understanding of these two categories of data collection as your choice about which you will use is closely related to the epistemology of methods and the perspective/analytic method you are using. Some approaches are able to appreciate the value of researcher-generated methods while others favour or even stipulate naturally occurring ones.

Researcher-generated methods create data that has been actively sought and created by the researcher. Researchers set-up an 'artificial' situation and generate data that would not otherwise have existed, by asking participants questions and recording their responses. The researcher creates an opportunity for data generation and the setting is thus contrived (Potter, 2002). If you refer to the literature on this discussion you will find that researcher-generated data collection methods are referred to by a number of terms including:

- Researcher-generated.
- Artificial.
- Contrived.
- Non-natural.

Naturally occurring data is data that would be generated (not necessarily recorded) without the researcher's involvement. In other words the interactions would occur whether the researcher was present or not. In this sense it is more 'natural'. Once a recording device is introduced to that natural setting and ethical procedures have been implemented, it becomes naturally occurring research, as the setting is still natural but the recording is for research purposes. As with researcher-generated data collection, naturally occurring data tends to be referred to in different ways in the literature, including terms such as:

- Naturally occurring.
- Natural.
- Naturalistic.

The dead social scientist test (Potter, 1996)

A useful way of differentiating between both types of data is to use the 'dead social scientist test'. This test questions whether the 'data' would still exist (not necessarily recorded) if the researcher was not able to collect it. A research interview or focus group would probably be cancelled if the researcher was not available to ask the questions. However, an interaction that was naturally occurring would still occur.

Example 1

An interview set up with a young child to talk about his experience of ADHD would be cancelled if the researcher was not able to attend.

Example 2

A video camera is routinely set up to record initial paediatric consultations with children with an autism diagnosis. If the researcher was not able to attend to collect the video material, the consultations would still go ahead.

Usually it is researchers who are practicing some types of discourse analysis or conversation analysis that prefer naturally occurring data and much of the debate regarding the value of naturally occurring data over researcher-generated tends to be promoted by those who favour these approaches.

> ### *A*   Activity   Naturally occurring or researcher-generated?
>
> If you are doing your own research project try to identify now whether you are collecting naturally occurring data or researcher-generated. In your research diary write down some of the reasons why this is suitable.

If you are still unsure then have a look at the flow chart in Figure 10.1.

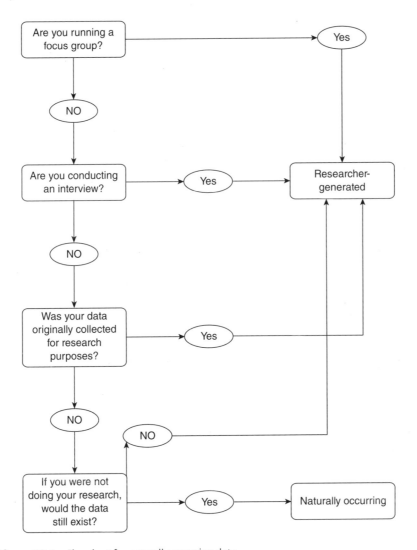

Figure 10.1   Flowchart for naturally occurring data

Outlining the debate

The debate regarding researcher-generated versus naturally occurring data collection focuses on the limits of the value of data collected using researcher-generated methods and the limits of using naturally occurring data. Typically the debate rests on two issues:

1. The influence of the researcher.
2. The ethical considerations.

There are researchers who argue that researcher-generated methods have a lot to offer child mental health, arguing that these methods can also be integrated with naturally occurring ones. Alternatively there are researchers who argue that researcher-generated methods only reflect the method itself and can be used as a topic of study but not to find something out.

 Some qualitative researchers caution that concerns about the distinctions between naturally occurring and researcher-generated data should not be taken too far (Silverman, 2006).

Historically children have been studied from a developmental or psychological perspective, using mostly quantitative and/or qualitative researcher-generated methods focusing on eliciting talk rather than exploring their natural conversations (Hamo et al., 2004). Arguably, however, exploring children in natural environments can provide a great deal of in-depth information that may be missed by researcher-generated approaches.

 Be clear about the type of data you want to collect and ensure that you have a sound rationale for your choice.

The first concern is the effect that you have on the data collection and research process. Some researchers seek to minimise this influence by gathering naturally occurring data as the researcher is less instrumental in the process. This is arguably problematic for the ethos of qualitative work and some have argued that by favouring naturally occurring data, researchers are contradicting a fundamental aspect of the paradigm and are in some sense viewing the researcher as one who contaminates the data (Speer, 2002). Of course this view is contentious and advocates of naturally occurring data do embrace the role of the researcher in the process but seek to explore children in their own natural worlds, rather than seeking it retrospectively through interviews (see Potter, 2002).

The second concern in the debate is ethics. There is a deliberate avoidance of calling data which has not been researcher-generated 'natural', favouring instead the notion of 'naturally occurring', to appreciate the influence of recording devices and the impact of implementing ethical principles. We do return to the influence of recording devices later in the book, but the focus of the discussion here relates to how the situation or event is altered by the introduction of a recording device. By recording the child mental health interaction and therefore turning it into 'data', and also by seeking consent from participants, the data could be argued to thus be partially contrived (Speer, 2002).

 Your choice between using naturally occurring data and researcher-generated data should depend on how you intend to study a particular phenomenon (Ten Have, 2002).

The naturally occurring interview

Just because you are collecting interview data does not automatically make it researcher-generated data, as naturally occurring interviews exist. The differentiation relates to how the data were collected and the purpose. If the interview was conducted for another purpose, other than research, it may fit the criteria for naturally occurring interview data. Naturally occurring interviews can be text-based, for example appearing in newspapers and magazines. They can also be verbal, for example with a presenter/news-reader asking an invited representative of an organisation questions with the answers being given in real time. We present two examples below.

Example 1   News interviews

These are naturally occurring interviews which are portrayed through the media, for example a health representative talking about government policies. The interviewer is not carrying out a research interview, but a news interview. This means that if you download or record the news interview for research purposes it has occurred naturally without your intervention. It passes the 'dead social scientist' test. News interviews can be a useful way of looking at how child mental health is represented in the media.

(Continued)

(Continued)

Example 2   Job interviews

These are also naturally occurring interviews. Recruitment interviewers question candidates for employment, and for your research you may choose to record these (ethics withstanding). These interviews again pass the 'dead social scientist' test. Recruitment interviews might be interesting to explore from a number of angles including recruitment of mental health staff, how personal mental health issues are accounted for in a job interview situation, or to look at teachers' proposed practical strategies for dealing with children with difficulties in the classroom.

Collecting naturally occurring data from clinical settings

While there are ethical sensitivities and practical challenges, obtaining naturally occurring data from clinical settings can produce rich data. If you look at the literature you will see that this type of data has been used well in general practice (Tates & Meeuwesen, 2000), paediatrics (Cahill & Papageorgiou, 2007), family therapy (O'Reilly & Parker, 2013b), child counselling (Hutchby, 2002) and mental health services (Antaki & O'Reilly, in press). This data type reveals additional issues about child mental health that may be missed by researcher-generated methods.

Challenges of collecting naturally occurring data from clinical settings

As our personal interests are in child mental health and language/interaction, we are experienced in collecting naturally occurring data from clinical settings. However, collecting this type of data does present challenges:

1. *Ethics.* You are asking to record vulnerable groups while they are undergoing a mental health intervention which is already bound up with issues of sensitivity and confidentiality. Thus there is additional sensitivity regarding the core ethical principles of informed consent, right to withdraw, confidentiality and debriefing.
2. *Potential perceived changes to clinical care.* Because you are recording the natural clinical context there is a risk that the children and their families may misunderstand the research. They may believe that their clinical care may be compromised if they refuse to participate, or may feel that their clinical care may be improved if they agree.

3. *Preparing families.* If you plan to record families or children in the institutional setting then you will need to give them time and advance notice of what to expect. To conform to ethical guidelines, families need to be prepared in advance that if they provide consent their session will be recorded. This should be done in writing and then on the day of the intervention this should be reiterated verbally.

4. *Gatekeepers.* The role of the gatekeeper is especially pertinent. If you ask to record the natural setting of therapy, psychiatry, counselling, education, social work and so forth, then you will also be recording those professionals doing their jobs. They may feel uncomfortable having their expertise put under such close scrutiny, may fear being judged/criticised, or may feel that you are intruding on a sensitive space.

5. *Practical recording issues.* To fully capture the natural environment it will require some equipment. In certain mental health environments people may move around the room. In some settings, some of the intervention occurs outside of the main room (for example, behind the one-way mirror in family therapy, or in some child assessments the child and parents may separate). If you are not prepared for this then you will miss some of the important interactions and decisions.

Personal case example: Overcoming the challenges

We have experiences of overcoming challenges of collecting naturally occurring data from clinical settings. There are no specific rules to follow as each situation will be different, but we provide you with general guidance. Our project required using video to record first assessment appointments at a Child and Adolescent Mental Health Service in the UK.

In relation to ethics – Not only will you have to think about the ethical issues invoked by recording a naturally occurring institutional event, but you will also need to convince the ethics committee that you have thought about why ethics are more sensitive with this type of data. This was important for us:

- We consulted with mental health professionals from different services across the UK, face-to-face and via email. We explained our plans and sought their advice. We invited comments on our proposal and asked lots of questions regarding potential obstacles (ethical and practical) they were able to foresee.
- We consulted several parents known to us through our professional networks and again invited comments. This gave us insight into how they might feel having their children recorded for research.

- We ensured that our research team was made up of clinical and academic professionals who had knowledge of mental health care and processes, organisational structures and methodological/ethical rigour.
- We attended the ethics committee meeting so that we could work with the ethics committee as a partner in our decision-making and discuss our concerns as well as those raised by the committee.

In relation to perceived changes – We acknowledged the risk of possible misconception and developed strategies to deal with this:

- First, we made sure this issue was attended to in our information sheets. We were transparent that participation or non-participation would _not_ affect their care and that the research team was separate from the clinical team.
- Second, a junior researcher took the consent to be less coercive. This researcher was not a clinician, did not work for the service from which data were collected and did not have a medical title.
- Finally, the clinical staff who participated in the research reassured families that the research made no difference to their care.

In relation to preparing families – We learned valuable lessons from consulting with families at the planning stage. In preparation for our video recording of the assessments we asked some families currently engaged with services what they thought about the project. We expected these families to be concerned with data protection, anonymity and the sensitivity of the session. However, they were able to see the benefits of the research. Surprisingly they seemed to mostly have concerns with how they may appear in the recording. Specific comments included:

- Consent should be taken on the day but advance notice given so that they could wear nice clothes for the video.
- Advance notice is important because one mother commented that she would like to wear make-up for the appointment if on video.
- Families reported that they liked the methodology and thought it would find interesting things.
- Families reported that they would be happy to be recorded for research like this as it is important to improve services.

In relation to gatekeepers – This can be tricky but is important. During planning we were aware that without the cooperation of the clinicians our project would fail. As we mentioned, we consulted with various clinical professionals known to us through our networks to get a general sense of how they felt and they gave us some ideas for approaching our potential participants. When we had identified a service and gained the agreement from clinical managers, we organised a meeting for a clinical member of our team to discuss the project with them. This allowed all potential participants to ask questions. At this point they were reassured that no judgements would be passed and that the transcripts would be anonymous.

In relation to recording issues – We were fortunate that the service recruited had recording equipment already installed. Permission was given to use this equipment. However, after recording the first two families we found that only one microphone had been plugged in so the sound quality was poor and that when one clinical professional left the room for an individual discussion with the child (separate from the family) that was not recorded. We learned two important lessons:

- First, to check the equipment through a dummy run.
- Second, we gave the clinical professionals a digital audio recorder to capture anything that occurred outside the main treatment room.

A   Activity   Think about your research project

After reading this case example, what have you learned that would help you improve your project? Make a list of people you could speak to who could give you feedback on your project that will enhance its likelihood of success.

Documents as data

Written texts are different from spoken language and the word 'text' is typically employed to mean the written document (Bryman, 2008). Documents are an important source of data in research (Drew, 2006) as much social life in contemporary society is mediated by written text (Atkinson & Coffey, 2004). Text-based documents such as official state documents, magazines, newspapers and transcripts of television programmes can be used as qualitative data (Bryman, 2008). Watson (1997) argues that the social world is loaded with documents which involve written language, indicating the immensely pervasive, institutionalised and widespread place of text in society. Watson lists many of these and we provide some of these suggestions below:

- Street signs.
- Public transport timetables.
- Company logos.
- Contracts.
- T-Shirt epigrams.
- Passports.

- Payslips.
- Greetings cards.
- Road markings and maps.
- Magazines and newspapers.

His list goes on to mention many more text-based documents but these examples should show how central documents are in our lives.

Using documents as data in child mental health can be a useful way of gaining insights into mental health organisations, mental health representations in the media and into children's lives. There are many different ways of using documents as data in child mental health, for example:

- Newspapers, magazines or internet pages in terms of how they represent child mental health conditions.
- Official policy or mental health organisational documents, such as policy documents, medical notes, meetings' minutes, staff email exchanges and official letters.
- Children's writings, such as diaries, letters, creative stories, poems and emails.
- Web-based blog/forum sites for parents and/or children to share personal experiences of particular mental health difficulties; social media sites.

Using existing documents such as those generated by the media or publicly available policy documents can give you some insight into how the public are informed about mental health issues. Analysing how different conditions are represented by newspapers or magazines can illustrate how the general public are influenced by publicly available notions of the disorders.

Organisations also represent mental health in different ways. These documents have the potential to reveal organisational structures, how understanding of patients is framed, how decisions are reached and how definitions or diagnosis of mental health conditions are negotiated. Organisations have ways of representing themselves and one of the characteristically contemporary social forms is through paperwork (Atkinson & Coffey, 2004).

 Be careful not to assume that documents reveal something about an underlying social reality, rather documents are a reality in their own right (Bryman, 2008).

If you do choose to analyse documents then be careful not to make assumptions regarding what they can reveal. Be aware that there is a danger in believing that the meaning is inscribed in the text itself and that you can discover what the writer intended through an analysis of the textual evidence (Widdowson, 2004). Texts are not a window to reality and do not represent a reality beyond the text (Watson, 1997). Try to remember that these documents are part of wider systems. This is known as 'intertextuality', a term from literary criticism which refers to the fact that texts are not free-standing, but are linked to other texts (Atkinson & Coffey, 2004).

A different way of using documents to explore child mental health is to analyse documents produced by children themselves. There are two ways to do this:

- First, you may choose to analyse children's documents, such as their short stories, diaries, letters, emails and so forth, that they have already produced as part of their education, their therapy/counselling, or their social development.
- Second, you can ask children to keep a diary over the course of time, ask them to produce stories or poems about something particular related to the research question, or ask them to communicate with you by letter or email.

The first type of documentary analysis is naturally occurring as the children are producing documents as part of their lives without your intervention. The second type of documents is researcher-generated as you have specifically asked the children to produce the documents for your research. Although there are lots of different documents produced by children we focus the rest of the chapter on diaries as they are a special form of qualitative data collection.

Diaries as data

Diaries are a useful way of understanding health/healthcare and can be especially helpful in understanding the context in which illnesses are experienced, needs expressed and accounts given (Elliott, 1997). Diary data is not common in qualitative research as there are many challenges to collecting it. Nonetheless diaries are useful in mental health research, particularly for therapy research (Mackrill, 2008). There are two main types of diary research:

1. *The solicited diary* – which is when a participant produces an account at the request of the researcher (Bell, 1998).
2. *The non-solicited diary* – are those that are written spontaneously by the participant and not directly for research purposes (Mackrill, 2008).

While the non-solicited diary can be a rich and insightful source of data it is especially difficult to obtain these entries as diaries are personal, intimate and private documents. Because of this, solicited diaries tend to be used with researchers asking children to keep a diary of their illness experiences. Diaries provide children a forum through which they are able to express themselves. To help you decide whether the solicited diary is a useful form of data collection for your own project we provide you with a table of advantages and disadvantages of the method in Table 10.1.

Table 10.1   The advantages and disadvantages of using solicited diaries

Advantages	Disadvantages
The diarists have control over what they reveal which means they may be willing to reveal more than through other methods (Mackrill, 2008).	Keeping a diary inevitably has an effect on participants' daily routines and potentially on their experiences (Willig, 2001).
Diaries can be useful in health research as events can be documented quickly after they occur which allows them to be examined (Butz & Alexander, 1991).	It can be difficult to encourage participants to participate in the study, particularly as motivation may wane if the study goes on too long (Butz & Alexander, 1991). This is especially true of child participants who can lose their motivation or attention.
Health diaries can be used to describe an array of chronic or short-term illnesses and can be used to collect information about an individual's health behaviours (Richardson, 1994).	There tend to be high drop-out rates in diary studies as participants lose interest in the research (Richardson, 1994).
Diaries are especially useful for exploring sensitive topics as sometimes participants feel more comfortable revealing things on paper than face-to-face (Mackrill, 2008).	There is a risk that participants may forget to fill in their diaries at the required times and may retrospectively fill in their entries (referred to as 'backfilling'), therefore relying on memory (Green et al., 2006).
Diaries provide access to very personal or intimate information which may not occur through other methods (Willig, 2001).	

If you decide that the solicited diary is useful then you need to plan effectively. We provide you with some practical suggestions before data collection:

- Formulate a clear set of instructions to guide participants (Willig, 2001).
- If participants have difficulty expressing themselves in writing you could ask them to make an audio recording of their diary entries instead (Jacelon & Imperio, 2005).
- It is important that you are clear regarding what kind and how much detail is expected in the entries (Willig, 2001).
- Although the most common approach to diary studies is to use pen and paper you may choose the option of using an electronic diary (Bolger et al., 2003), which has the benefit of electronic reminders or more interactive/creative ways of writing (Green et al., 2006).

> ## *A*   Activity   Diary practice
>
> For one week, set yourself the challenge of writing your own personal health diary. Give yourself a clear set of guidelines. Try to complete the diary at the same time each day. At the end of the week, discuss your experience with a friend or colleague and assess your views on the value and potential obstacles of this method of data collection.

Summary

This chapter has introduced you to the considerations important in thinking about the differences between researcher-generated and naturally occurring data. Here we have also provided you with guidance for differentiating the two types of data collection, whilst illustrating the central features of the debate in the literature. The chapter concluded with a focus on documents as data, considering their value for child mental health research and making decisions as to the appropriate types of documents to study.

Key messages

- For data to be considered naturally occurring, it must pass the 'dead researcher' test.
- Collecting naturally occurring data from clinical settings poses additional practical and ethical challenges.
- Documents are a useful and interesting form of child mental health data and come in many forms.
- Diary data provides valuable insights into children's health experiences.

Further reading

Butz, A. & Alexander, C. (1991). Use of health diaries with children. *Nursing Research*, 40(1), 59–61.

Drew, P. (2006). When documents 'speak': documents, language and interaction. In P. Drew, G. Raymond & D. Weinberg (eds), *Talk and interaction in social research methods* (pp. 63–80). London: Sage.

Potter, J. (2002). Two kinds of natural. *Discourse Studies*. 4(4), 539–542.

CHAPTER 11

INTERNET METHODS

Learning outcomes

- Appreciate the need to safeguard children on the internet.
- Recognise the challenges and benefits of recruiting online.
- Differentiate the different forms of online data collection methods.
- Identify the main ethical issues with this type of research.

Introduction

Researchers are now relying more on the internet for recruiting participants and collecting data. When conducting child mental health
research, this method has potential benefits and you may decide that

this is a cost-effective way of doing your research. In this chapter we provide you with the tools and information to carry out internet-based methods effectively with children. Children's use of the internet raises some safeguarding issues and these are well documented in relation to general usage. Some of these issues have implications for child research and are thus addressed in this chapter.

You may choose to use the internet to recruit your participants and then use traditional face-to-face methods of data collection or you may recruit through traditional methods and then use internet technology to collect the data. Alternatively you may choose to recruit and collect your data online. These different modalities have several benefits and challenges and this chapter will help you plan effectively. The chapter concludes with some additional discussion of ethics as online methods provoke additional and sometimes different ethical sensitivities to those already discussed.

Safeguarding children in the digital age

To appreciate child research in the online context it is first important to look at the broader issue of children and internet use as a platform for discussion. We now live in a digital information age and children are living in a world filled with technology. The developing and evolving range of technologies mean that children need to have knowledge to use these pieces of high-tech equipment (Ahmedani et al., 2011). An important technological advancement for children has been access to the internet. Internet access has generally increased as many children in many countries now have access to the internet at home (Valke et al., 2011). Indeed most children could not conceive of their lives without technology (Ahmedani et al., 2011).

Typical internet usage for children tends to follow three dimensions, entertainment, education and edutainment (Livingstone, 2003), with the fourth added as consumerism, as children begin engaging in e-commerce (Tufte, 2006). This increased engagement with and different dimensions of internet usage, however, can pose risks for children and it is important you appreciate those specific to the research context. The internet poses risks for children as it contains content which is linked with violence, pornography, racism or hate (Valke, et al., 2011) and there is no simple solution for protecting children online (Sharples et al., 2009). This is concerning when research shows that young people seem more willing than other groups to post personal information, with up to 70% revealing their name, telephone number, age, address and other personal details (Sharples et al., 2009).

Activity   Relevance to research

How do you think these issues affect the research context? Why might general safeguarding issues matter in the online research context?

Society traditionally relies on parents for safeguarding children from the potentially harmful effects of the media (Wartella & Jennings, 2000) but in your role as a researcher you will also have a part to play in this protection in the context of your project. General safeguarding issues matter, as parents are sensitive to adult strangers 'lurking' on the internet targeting children. Although your intentions are (hopefully) good, children and their parents need to understand that you are credible and not a criminal posing as a researcher.

Recruiting through the internet

Recruiting online has benefits and challenges. You may find it useful at this point to refer to Chapter 6 on recruitment, as much of that information applies to the online context too. We noted in that chapter that it is important that you recruit an adequate and representative sample, but sometimes there are barriers to getting access to children. Researchers therefore may turn to the internet to recruit vulnerable populations when they encounter these barriers from institutions (Cook, 2011).

Recruiting participants through the internet, however, is less well established than other methods with some concerns regarding the representativeness of online samples (Koo & Skinner, 2005). It is generally recognised that those with internet access broadly reflect the general population but it is important that you remain mindful of the changing demographics of internet users and how this may influence the usefulness of internet recruitment for your study (Hamilton & Bowers, 2006). Furthermore there are issues of access and the overwhelming amount of information posted online. If you post an advertisement on the internet to recruit children and families, reaching them may be difficult and therefore you will really need to think about how you target your participants. Nonetheless research shows that people are turning to the internet to find out more about their health conditions and therefore it is possible for potential participants to readily find research advertisements (Cook, 2011).

 It is important that you consider your sampling method before you begin recruitment.

Through email

Email can be a useful medium for recruiting participants. Many children use email to communicate and have email addresses. Often it is possible to obtain email lists and send out one group email, although this may be more difficult to access with children than with adults. Remember that it is probable that you will first have to email parents to secure their interest before you can email children directly. It is helpful if in your email to the child and parent you include a hyperlink to the project website so that they can find out more information about your study (Koo & Skinner, 2005).

There are a number of things you can do to help increase the likelihood that participants will respond. Meho (2006) provides some general guidance:

- Make sure you write something in the subject line to reduce the likelihood that the email will be ignored or deleted.
- Be succinct regarding your request.
- Be professional.
- Make sure you are clear about ethics.

It is helpful if you can send personal email invitations to individual parents and children rather than a group email which simply outlines the project. This will have a more personal feel. By referring to them by name in the email they are less likely to view it as SPAM.

 Do not allow all email addresses to be visible if sending a group email, not all parents/children will want this information shared; use the bcc option or send separate emails.

Through online discussion boards

A useful way to recruit children is to use discussion boards. These can be especially helpful if you are targeting specific groups of children. Often there are peer support groups online for particular disorders or for families of children who have a mental health difficulty. You can use these discussion boards and forums to post a link to your research project website. Some of these virtual groups will have membership lists which may help you to establish a sampling frame, but note that not all of these organisations will allow you access to these lists (Wright, 2005).

Some messages may be removed by board administrators if they are perceived as SPAM or if they violate discussion board rules (Koo & Skinner, 2005).

Typically, accessing populations through the use of discussion boards, chat rooms or community bulletin boards is achieved by posting invitations to the website (Hudson & Bruckman, 2004). If you are going to recruit this way then you will need to pay particular attention to how you word your advertisement and think about the language you use in it. It is helpful to give your advertisement a clear title and provide simple explanations.

 Some members of the online community may find your advertisement or intrusion of their space offensive or rude (Hudson & Bruckman, 2004).

Summarising internet recruitment

To summarise, there are many ways to improve your recruitment online and Meho (2006) provides some useful tips:

- It is better to solicit participants individually rather than through message boards or mailing lists.
- Write something in the 'subject line' to reduce the likelihood of your message being deleted.
- Make sure you introduce yourself properly in the message and provide some details of your credibility.
- Tel them how their email address or other information was acquired as this promotes trust.
- Be open and honest about your research, its aims and purpose.
- Give the potential participants information regarding what types of questions to expect, how much of their time is required and how many times they will be contacted.
- Outline any possible benefits of taking part.
- Respond quickly to any questions or queries.

Data collection online

There are different ways to collect data through the internet. Many traditional methods of data collection such as questionnaires, interviews and naturally occurring data can be employed in an online modality.

Questionnaires/surveys

Perhaps the most common form of data collection online is surveys/questionnaires, which tend to be quantitative. This is where the child will sit at a computer and provide their answers electronically. Internet questionnaires are also known as computerised self-administered questionnaires (Norman et al., 2001). The technology for internet-based research is evolving and the development of software packages are making online questionnaire research much easier (Wright, 2005). Software such as SurveyMonkey allows the researcher to design a questionnaire online and then distribute it widely to large samples of children.

There are different ways of designing your internet questionnaire and you need to think about how to encourage children to complete all of the questions. Three main designs have been considered by Norman et al. (2001):

1. You can design one long continuous document that requires the child to scroll down through the questions meaning they can see the whole questionnaire in one go. This may, however, confuse some children.
2. You can design your questionnaire so only one question or section is presented at a time. This helps the child to focus on a single question but may lose the context of the design.
3. You can provide semantic indexes where the child navigates through questions in a linear manner.

Whichever design style you choose be mindful of the way in which you write your questions, the language you use and the length of time children need to complete all questions. You might want to refer back to the section on questionnaires in Chapter 8 as much of the guidance for developing postal or face-to-face questionnaires applies here. In that chapter we outlined the advantages and disadvantages of using questionnaires with children, however, using the internet as a tool for data collection has additional benefits and limitations, some of which are listed in Table 11.1.

Although using internet questionnaires can be useful, perhaps the most problematic concern for child mental health research is age. Participants who are responding to these requests may misrepresent their age, gender or level of education (Wright, 2005) and therefore you may not truly be getting answers from children, or from the age group of children you are targeting. You may therefore find it is useful to replicate your questionnaire with a different group of children to gain a reliable picture of the characteristics of online questionnaire participants (Wright, 2005).

Table 11.1   The advantages and disadvantages of using internet questionnaires with children

Advantages	Disadvantages
Internet questionnaires have the potential to be more interactive (Norman et al., 2001). This can make them more interesting and appealing for children.	You cannot be sure that the answers are honest or the participants are who they say they are (Wright, 2005).
The use of internet questionnaires helps the researcher to reach participants in distant locations (Wright, 2005).	The design space of an internet questionnaire is enormous and it is easy to get confused or have technical problems. The interface development must be guided by the research and reasoned principles (Norman et al., 2001).
Most institutions have sufficient internet access which means that there is little extra cost to present the questionnaire in this way; thus internet questionnaires are more cost effective than postal or face-to-face (Fox et al., 2003).	There may be some issues over sampling and the representativeness of the sample as only internet users can fill in the questionnaire (Fox et al., 2003).
There is a greater speed of administration with internet questionnaires than postal or face-to-face (Schmidt, 1997).	There may be concerns regarding the validity and reliability of the data produced by this method (Wright, 2005).
There are some cases where particular groups or communities only exist in cyberspace and these virtual communities offer a mechanism to access those beliefs, interests and values on a particular issue (Wright, 2005).	

Synchronous and asynchronous methods

There are many different ways of collecting qualitative data online, with the most common being interviews and focus groups. This means there are choices of how to interview children using the internet, or how to run your focus groups. Interviews conducted over the internet tend to fall into one of two categories, asynchronous and synchronous. Asynchronous are those which are computer-mediated and remain text-based (Stewart & Williams, 2005). These do not require the researcher and participant to be using the internet at the same time (Hunt & McHale, 2007). Synchronous methods are those that require the researcher and the participant to be using the internet at the same time and this can be done through text or verbally (Jowett et al., 2011). We present the alternative methods in Table 11.2.

Table 11.2   Asynchronous and synchronous methods

Asynchronous	Synchronous
Email	Skype
Discussion boards	Instant messaging
Blogs	Chat rooms
Social networking sites	

When conducting interviews using the internet, it may be text-based or verbal. This form of interviewing can enable vulnerable populations, such as children with mental health difficulties, to participate (Cook, 2011) and can provide good opportunities for researching families (Berger & Paul, 2011). There are, however, some limitations to using the internet to conduct interviews or focus groups and you may need either to minimise these before you start, or take them into account in the discussion of your findings:

- Online interviewing can lack visual cues and other cues such as tone of voice which typically facilitate communication (Jowett et al., 2011) particularly with children, or those with communication impairments.
- Internet communication is sometimes regarded as a more detached, impersonal and impoverished form of social communication (Hewson et al., 1996).
- Online interviewing can require more time from you than traditional face-to-face interviews (Jowett et al., 2011).
- Different family members are more or less familiar with technology which may create some risk of inequity among the family members in terms of having their voices heard (Berger & Paul, 2011).
- There may be technological difficulties as computers may crash, power cuts may occur or internet connections may be lost (Jowett et al., 2011).
- Online communication has its own forms of paralanguage such as abbreviations (lol = laugh-out-loud), emoticons (☺) or asterisks to denote bodily actions (*grin*) and it can be difficult to decipher this local language or ascertain whether participants are happy or uncomfortable with your line of questions (Jowett et al., 2011).

Despite the various problems that may occur in the online interview it is still considered to be a useful method for accessing vulnerable or hard-to-reach populations and can save resources. What will matter is how you manage these limitations in practice.

Using email

Email is a common form of communication, but its value as an interviewing technique has not been fully assessed (Hunt & McHale, 2007). The asynchronous nature of email interviewing can be useful for obtaining children's views or experiences. Email can facilitate communication, particularly for those with disabilities as often these individuals find the internet a useful modality for social interaction (Ison, 2009). Using email may encourage disclosure of sensitive topics (Cook, 2011) and offers flexibility in terms of convenience, timing and geography (Ison, 2009). There are some important things you need to consider if you are going to use this medium with children and Table 11.3 provides some advice.

Table 11.3 Practical tips for using email methods with children

Tip	Description
Allow sufficient time (Meho, 2006).	It may take some children time to respond to your email questions, so be patient, but do follow up if you feel it is necessary.
Communicate that you are listening (O'Connor & Madge, 2001).	It is important that you promote a positive experience and therefore giving regular feedback and assurances can be helpful.
Start with broad questions (Ison, 2009).	It can be helpful to start off with broad and general questions, particularly for those with mental health difficulties. Do not ask too much in any single question.
Check the meanings in the data (Cook, 2011).	Use the on-going nature of the email exchange to check meanings in the data and reflect on what has been said.
Reiterate the content of the previous email (Ison, 2009).	It can be useful to reflect back on what the child said in the previous email to you.
Think about the number of questions you ask (Burns, 2010).	Be careful not to ask too many questions in any single email. Keep your questions simple and understandable and give the children the opportunity to ask you what a question means if they do not understand.
You can conduct more than one interview at a time (Hunt & McHale, 2007).	Do not restrict yourself to conducting one interview at a time as email exchanges can take several days. It may take you weeks to get all of your questions answered.

While we have considered the benefits of using email to interview children with mental health difficulties, it is important that you are aware of some of the limitations of this method so that, where possible, you can reduce these problems:

- Email interviews may take a long time to conduct and there is a risk that the participant's enthusiasm may reduce (Hunt & McHale, 2007). Some children with mental health difficulties may also have physical disabilities. It is important to note that for some their physical disability prevents them from typing on a computer and there is a risk of excluding them from your study (Ison, 2009).
- The lack of personal contact may be viewed adversely by some participants (James & Busher, 2006).
- Some participants may not be able to articulate as effectively through text as they can verbally (Karchmer, 2001).

Remember then, if you are going to use email to interview children you need to build rapport and hold their attention. In a typical face-to-face interview you will only require the participant to attend for a short time – 30 minutes to 2 hours – but email interviews can take place over a long period of time. It might therefore be helpful to set some time limits on the interview, have a clear end date and set dates for when each question needs to be answered (Hunt & McHale, 2007). It will be important that you agree these with the child before the interview starts.

Using Instant Messaging

Instant Messaging is a synchronous form of computer-mediated conversation and one that is commonly used amongst younger generations (Fontes & O'Mahony, 2008). As this is a medium of communication which is popular amongst young people it has potential to be a useful way of interviewing children with mental health difficulties. Although some children will be more familiar with the technology than others, and the country of origin of the child may make a difference to this familiarity, it could be a useful way for you to obtain their views. Instant messaging software tends to alert you to when the participant is typing a message and this reduces the likelihood of interruptions (Hinchcliffe & Gavin, 2009) and it also alerts you to inactivity. It is important to remember, however, that children are developing academically and some children, especially younger children, may have some difficulty articulating their views or may worry about spelling and grammar. As with other methods there are some clear advantages to using this modality with children and some limitations. We provide an overview of these in Table 11.4.

Table 11.4   The advantages and disadvantages of using Instant Messaging

Advantages	Disadvantages
It can be a useful method for those with communication difficulties or hearing impairments (Hinchcliffe & Gavin, 2009).	Instant Messaging interviews take longer than face-to-face ones (Hinchcliffe & Gavin, 2009).
The communication occurs in real time which makes the interview more conversation like than some other text-based methods (Flynn, 2004).	Interviewees have time to consider their answers and may censor some of their responses (O'Connor & Madge, 2001).
Instant Messaging has the capacity to generate reflective and descriptive data (James & Busher, 2006).	Taking field notes during the interview is an important part of the process but this can be more difficult when typing at the same time (Opdenakker, 2006).
It is possible to archive and store conversations (Flynn, 2004).	Terminating an Instant Messaging interview can be quite difficult and may feel abrupt (Opdenakker, 2006).

 Do not forget that your decision to use Instant Messaging (or any other method) should be driven by the advantages and limitations, but more importantly by your research question.

Using Skype

There have been advancements in technology which now mean you may enjoy the benefits of online interviewing, but have the additional advantage of the interview being face-to-face. This can be especially useful with children as you will be able to hold their attention more effectively and undertake the interview in real time. Skype interviewing provides a forum for cutting the costs of calls and is a simple way to communicate through video-chat (Bertrand & Bordeau, 2010). Many children are familiar with Skype and have their own Skype account or can use the account of their parents. As a researcher you can use the Skype-to-Skype virtual interaction to record interviews and collect both verbal and non-verbal data (Evans et al., 2008).

Although ostensibly this may seem a strong method of data collection as it has many of the benefits of transcending distance and ability, it is important to appreciate the limitations of a Skype-to-Skype interview. Remember not all children will be comfortable talking to a computer screen and there is still the potential that they will become distracted by what is going on around them in their own environment. There are also questions about whether the data produced is reliable and valid, and non-verbal communication cannot be used in quite the same way as traditional face-to-face (Bertrand & Bordeau, 2010). To be able to use this medium some children will need to set up a Skype profile page to be able to participate in your research and you may need to provide some technological support for families to enable them to do this.

Using discussion boards, blogs and chat rooms

Discussion boards, blogs and chat rooms provide you with a different kind of data. They are not researcher-led in that you will not be necessarily asking questions directly to participants, but rather the text is already being created by children in cyberspace and you are using that as data. This sharing and connecting of people through the internet is traditionally referred to as Web 2.0 (Tapscott & Williams, 2008). We differentiate these different modalities in Table 11.5.

It is obvious that these three forms of text-based online discussions are similar to each other and are likely to attract child members. Blogs and chat rooms are similar as they both allow the researcher to participate in and observe textual conversations. Blogs can be a useful form of internet data on children as they can offer insights into their health and illness experiences (Eastham, 2011). Blogs are like personal diaries and these can be shared publicly if the blogger allows it (Chenail, 2011). As blogging is becoming more popular it is offering a useful mechanism for data collection as blogs are low cost and publicly available (Hookway, 2008).

Table 11.5 Discussion boards, blogs and chat rooms

Medium	Description
Discussion board	A discussion board is an online modality which allows groups to discuss ideas with each other. It creates a number of 'threads' which can be responded to by members of the group.
Blogs	Blogs are text-based entries onto a website that consist of personal or professional narratives and may be accompanied by pictures or video (Eastham, 2011).
Chat rooms	The primary purpose of chat rooms is to share information with others. This chat tends to occur in real time, rather than being asynchronous like discussion boards.

Hookway (2008) argues that there are four practical steps to using blogs as data:

1. You need to locate the blogs. Most blogs are hosted by blog content management systems and therefore you will need to engage in an initial scoping exercise.
2. You will then need to sample. Most blog content management systems have a search feature which will allow you to find bloggers according to demographic information such as age.
3. You will then need to establish an online presence to enter the worlds of those participants.
4. Once you have considered any ethical issues, you can then collect data in two phases. The passive phase of blog trawling and the active phase of blog solicitation.

You will need to be mindful though that when blog entries are uploaded onto a content management system they are protected by copyright which means that the blogger has exclusive rights over the reproduction of their work and this may be a limiting issue for you (Hookway, 2008).

Using social networking sites

With the advancement of social networking there is now greater interest in tapping into this as data. Social networking sites can provide a database of children that is vastly larger than other modalities (Moreno et al., 2008). Social media moderating includes the observation of social networking sites such as Facebook, Twitter and MySpace (Branthwaite & Patterson, 2011), with perhaps the most common being Facebook. Facebook was launched in 2004 and allows the personal profiles of individuals to be viewed by members of that network (Lewis et al., 2008). Facebook allows the profile owner to create an online page which includes personal information and to communicate with other profile owners (Moreno et al., 2012). Facebook has an advantage of allowing the researcher to study posts by an individual over the course of several months or years to look at changes over time (Paulus et al., 2014).

Research on older children shows that as many as 97.4% of 1640 students had a Facebook page (Lewis et al., 2008), which indicates that it could be a lucrative source of data. To systematically collate data taken from social networking sites is referred to as web-scraping or web-harvesting (Paulus et al., 2014). If you choose to use this as a source of data you need to consider how social media users oscillate between the world of social media and the real world (Branthwaite & Patterson, 2011). Remember that children will act out their social lives on Facebook quite differently to in their real worlds (Lewis et al., 2008). The social media world can be impractical, self-indulging, superficial, transient and identity driven (Branthwaite & Patterson, 2011).

 Activity   Facebook data

Think about how you might lift data from a Facebook page. Open up your own Facebook page now (if you don't have one ask a relative/ friend). What do you think is the best way of physically taking data from profile pages so that you might code or analyse the material?

One way of taking data from social networking sites is simply to copy and paste the materials into a word document. It is fairly simple to highlight the status posts that you wish to study and any pictures that accompany them and paste them into a Word page. A more efficient method, however, may be to work with a computer programmer to develop a data-mining algo-rithm which can detect the type of internet pages desired (Paulus et al., 2014). While this is a better method as it allows finding and cutting of the information you want, it may require payment or expertise that you do not have access to. It may be helpful to seek technical support from your insti-tution to see what expertise is available.

Ethics of online research

Ethical concerns are just as important with this online research as with other types which involve children. If you plan to study communities online this will create new ethical concerns and you should plan for this at the start of your study (Paulus et al., 2014). While for some forms of research with children over the internet it may be obvious what the ethical boundaries are, for others it may be blurred.

Example

If you have recruited children in order to carry out interviews/focus groups with them through Skype, email or Instant Messaging, then like any other form of interview you will need to obtain consent at a number of levels, offer the right to withdraw, debrief them and assure anonymity and confidentiality.

Example

If you are taking data from social networking sites, chat rooms, discussion boards, online support groups, blogs or other available internet sources then the ethical boundaries are blurred. There are some contentions regarding whether these constitute publicly accessible or private data.

Research on the internet is too broad for a single approach to ethics and you need to consider the unique risks and benefits that your research raises (Herring, 1996). For our discussion of ethics we focus on the modalities where the boundaries are blurred, rather than online interviews where there is much more clarity regarding consent and confidentiality. What is important to bear in mind is the potential for harm.

 Harm can still occur in internet research and it is more difficult to do anything to help when it does occur (Convery & Cox, 2012).

The potential for harm, however, in this kind of research can be unclear and may arise in unanticipated ways; it is important to plan ahead and discuss plans with your ethics committee (Hudson & Bruckman, 2004). There are some important questions you need to ask yourself when undertaking research with children online.

Do you need to obtain parental and child consent?

When making the decision whether to obtain consent from the children and parents for your study you must first determine whether the information you are gathering is considered 'public' or 'private'. This dichotomy however, is not as straightforward as it may first appear. You cannot assume that just because the information is accessible publicly that the individuals who posted it up intended it to be publicly visible (Eysenbach & Till, 2001).

Problems for social networking sites

Although research exploring the ethics of research on the internet is fairly new we are beginning to develop an understanding of the unique challenges that studying social networking sites pose for researchers. This of course is considerably more complex when the participants are under the age of 18. Additionally, if you are studying child mental health then your topic is likely to be more sensitive and this in itself makes your research more ethically challenging. Before you read ahead to the ethical problems related to social networking research attempt an answer for the following activity.

Case study

Tasia is training to be an occupational therapist and has an interest in drug and alcohol addiction. Tasia wants to explore how alcohol use is portrayed by older children on social networking sites and comes to you (as her supervisor) with a draft of her ethics application. On this application she has written that there are no ethical concerns because the data is publicly accessible.

A   **Activity   Helping Tasia**

What advice would you give Tasia?

As we have already noted there are issues with the private/public dichotomy and doing research online does raise some ethical issues which Tasia needs to account for. Undertaking research with children through social networking sites raises some specific challenges and we consider some of these in Table 11.6.

Although some research has been conducted on social networking sites such as Facebook and MySpace without obtaining the consent of the participants, this is potentially a risky strategy, particularly with child participants. The bottom line is, if in doubt, obtain consent and discuss the matter in depth with your ethics committee and research team/supervisor.

Table 11.6   Ethical challenges of social networking site research

Challenge	Description
Intended for a private audience (Moreno et al., 2008).	Although some children may understand that some of the information can be accessed more publicly it is likely to be intended for the private audience of their 'friends' network and it is disrespectful to treat it as public data.
Friends and networks restrict access (Zimmer, 2010).	If you are on the network or 'friends' list of a particular child then you can access their page and you may not realise the privacy settings of that child which restrict the view. This means that you may be mistaken into thinking the data is public when it is not.
Assessing the child's capacity (Moreno et al., 2008).	Central to obtaining consent from children is competence and capacity. It can be especially difficult to ascertain whether the child has capacity from the information on a social networking site, although there will be important clues there. The child may include their age, level of education, and from their posts you may yield some sense of their reasoning skills and language ability.
Unauthorised secondary use of personal information (Zimmer, 2010).	It is possible that using Facebook data without consent from the child could be considered unauthorised secondary use of personal information. This is because the information is collected on the page for a particular purpose and to use it for a different, secondary purpose is unauthorised without consent.

Problems for chat rooms, discussion boards and blogs

Ostensibly chat rooms, discussion boards and blogs may seem more public than social networking sites as it is very easy to enter a chat room, contribute to a discussion board or read a blog. Notably, however, research informs us that typically individuals in chat rooms do not approve of being researched and voice some strong objections to the presence of researchers (Hudson & Bruckman, 2004). This implies that the ethicality of this kind of research is more sensitive than believed and is something you should consider in more detail if you are going to use them as a modality for your project. We present some of the practical considerations in Table 11.7.

It can be quite confusing deciding whether you need to obtain consent to use blogs, chat rooms or discussion boards but some common sense is helpful. Where possible it is helpful to obtain consent or at least assent to use the data and look for signs that your presence is welcome or unwelcome. Most importantly do not assume the data is public and usable automatically.

How do you manage confidentiality/anonymity of online data?

Maintaining the anonymity of your participants and protecting confidentiality is important. This is equally important in online research but poses

Table 11.7   Practical ethical considerations for chat rooms, blogs and discussion boards

Consideration	Solution
Explore whether membership is needed for the site (Mayer & Till, 1996).	If membership is needed to subscribe to the site then it is feasible that writers are likely to regard the space as more private. You could use this benchmark to decide whether to seek consent from the contributing children or not.
Announcing your presence (Hudson & Bruckman, 2004)	One way of managing the consent issue is to announce your presence on the discussion board or chat room so that participants know you are there and can choose to 'opt in' by making contributions or 'opt out' be leaving the forum.
Hostility on the site (Eysenbach & Till, 2001).	There is a risk that the participants become hostile to your intrusion and therefore may stop engaging in the support group or discussion board which was originally helping them. This may then inadvertently cause them harm. You could set up your own chat room for the research and post a link on the original saying you will not visit it again, but those interested parties can go to your chat room.
Old but accessible data (Holmes, 2009).	Some conversations from discussion boards and chat rooms remain accessible for years after they have been posted and it could be practically impossible to trace the participant for consent. You are then faced with the choice of determining whether it is public or private data. If you consider it private then you should not use it.
Attempts at reducing access (Eastham, 2011).	Some bloggers and chat rooms attempt privacy by limiting access and this is a clear indication that they wish the material to be private. It should therefore be treated as such.
The role of the moderator (Hudson & Bruckman, 2004).	Many chat rooms and discussion boards have a moderator who has the ability to control the features of the conversation and remove unwanted individuals (such as researchers) from the site. It may be useful to identify the moderator and discuss your research with them before starting your research.

slightly different challenges to other methods. There are some benefits in relation to anonymity which include:

- The greater degree of anonymity with some online methods, such as online interviewing, can mean that the child feels less inhibited discussing sensitive issues (Jowett et al., 2011).
- Some forms of online text, such as blogs or chat rooms, allow the writer to adopt a pseudo-identity which means that their real identity is not revealed to you as a researcher (Eastham, 2011).
- Stigmatised populations may be more likely to contribute to research in which they feel their identity is masked by anonymity (Jowett et al., 2011).

While you might think that internet research affords a greater degree of anonymity to participants it is important to remember that this is not necessarily the case. You have a responsibility to protect the anonymity of the children who participate in your research and recognise the limits of confidentiality. There are a number of things you need to bear in mind before you collect your data:

- In many internet spaces, such as social networking sites, children will use their real names and identities (Paulus et al., 2014).
- IP addresses can be traced back to individual computers so despite a pseudonym you may still be able to find out the identity of the writer (Nosek et al., 2002).
- Just because names are removed from a chat room does not mean it is not possible to identify the children from other identifying information (Convery & Cox, 2012).
- Children particularly are likely to post personal details, addresses and photographs on the internet (Lenhart & Madden, 2007).
- Even if you anonymise social networking data there is a risk of deductive disclosure. This means that from the details in the post the participant may be identified by those who know them (Zimmer, 2010).
- Chat or Instant Messaging online risks being intercepted by a third party, although there are more secure encrypted chat software devices available (Ayling & Mewse, 2009).

 Simply removing the names from what you quote in your research may not be enough to protect the child's identity.

Summary

In this chapter we have introduced you to some of the general concerns regarding children's use of the internet and considered what these safeguarding issues mean for researchers. There are many different ways of recruiting and studying children online and we have provided you with some practical guidance relating to these. In this chapter we have given you some practical tips for carrying out internet-based research and considered some of the benefits and limitations of each of those approaches. This chapter has concluded with some discussion of the unique ethical sensitivities which are pertinent to the online approach.

Key messages

- The internet is being more widely used by children and more children have access now to a computer than before.
- Recruiting children through the internet can facilitate recruitment of children from diverse populations and from geographically inaccessible locations.

(Continued)

(Continued)

- There are a range of online modalities for collecting data including email, Skype, Instant Messaging, social networking sites, chat rooms, discussion boards and blogs.
- Some of the ethical sensitivities raised are different in online research and these relate mostly to whether the data is public or private.

Further reading

Evans, A., Elford, J. & Wiggins, S. (2008). Using the internet for qualitative research. In C. Willig & W. Stainton-Rogers (eds), *The Sage handbook of qualitative research in psychology* (pp. 315–333). London: Sage.

Lenhart, A. & Madden, M. (2007). *Teens, privacy and online social networks: How teens manage their online identities and personal information in the age of MySpace*. Washington DC: Pew Internet and American Life Project.

Paulus, T., Lester, J. N. & Dempster, P. (2014). *Digital tools for qualitative research*. London: Sage.

CHAPTER 12

RECORDING AND TRANSCRIPTION

Learning outcomes

- Review the value of audio and video recording in qualitative research.
- Recognise the challenges of using video for health research.
- Assess the arguments related to transcription.
- Debate the issues related to employing a transcriptionist.

Introduction

Most forms of qualitative research rely on recording the data. Typically you need to decide whether to record your data using audio or video equipment. In this chapter we guide you through some of the important decisions you need to make about your recording equipment and explore why video materials are becoming more popular in health research. Specifically we investigate some of the arguments regarding the effect recording equipment has on children in the research context and differentiate some of the issues that are integral to child mental health research decisions.

The second part of the chapter focuses on the issues relating to transcribing the recorded materials. We consider transcription an active process and guide you through decisions relating to the different conventions of transcription notation. We illustrate some issues pertinent to children's talk and also consider the matter of translation from other languages. We conclude the chapter with some consideration of the use of paid transcriptionists and the implications that this has for ethics and research quality.

Audio versus video

Clearly there have been technological advancements recently and the rise of digital equipment has been welcomed in research. Digital technology has offered great diversity in how you can present your findings and allows for the creation of clips, still frames and transcribed text (Miles, 2006). When you plan your research study you will need to make a decision whether to audio record your data or video record it.

 Whichever modality you choose, make sure that you are familiar with your recording device and know where all of the buttons are and what function they serve.

Think about the benefits and limitations of each and weigh these up in relation to your time, resources and research question. We start by comparing the benefits and limitations of audio recording in Table 12.1 and then do the same for video recording in Table 12.2.

Table 12.1 The benefits and limitations of audio

Benefits	Limitations
Audio equipment can be picked up fairly cheaply and is cost-effective (Gibbs et al., 2002).	You cannot capture non-verbal gestures which may be important in analysis.
It is possible your recruitment rates will be higher if you are audio recording than if you are video recording (Themessl-Huber et al., 2008).	Audio recordings do not allow you to see the context in which the interaction takes place and there is a risk that you may misinterpret something that has been said by a child.
Audio allows you to get close to your participants without them feeling as though their space is being intruded.	When there are multiple parties present it can sometimes be difficult when listening to the recording to differentiate between them.

Table 12.2   The benefits and limitations of video

Benefits	Limitations
Video allows you to access all verbal and non-verbal behaviour (Grimshaw, 1982).	Video equipment is typically more expensive than audio, but the prices are lowering.
Video can be a useful tool for practitioners to make sense of their interactions with children (Grimandi, 2007).	The use of video raises additional ethical sensitivities and is subject to additional scrutiny by ethics committees who may question your rationale for using it.
Video is especially useful for collecting naturally occurring data as it allows the whole context to be explored (Heath, 2004).	Your field of vision may be limited and you may need more than one camera to capture the full setting, thus being more expensive.

A   **Activity   Choosing a device**

After considering the benefits and limitations of audio and video, which do you think is most suitable for your research? Try to write a five-line rationale for your decision in your research diary.

Of course there are some benefits and limitations common to both modalities and it is important that you take these into account when planning:

- There is a permanence to the recording which allows you to refer to the data long after it has been collected, although there will be some ethical restrictions on this.
- Digital modalities allow you to edit, disguise and manipulate sounds and images which may be useful for presenting research (Gibbs et al., 2002).
- Both forms are easy to operate and have simple, safe ways of storing the data securely.
- You will need to ensure that you get good sound quality and consider where you place the microphones/cameras.
- Background noise can be intrusive when you come to later analyse the data and may prevent you from hearing some important information.

   Whether you choose audio or video remember to test for clarity and quality and consider issues such as the placement of the camera/microphone (Bottorff, 1994).

Choosing a recording device

When you have decided which modality to use it is necessary to think about the equipment itself. If you are doing a small-scale project and not likely to need it again, it is better to borrow equipment from your institution. If you are going to regularly undertake research it can be worth investing in some quality equipment of your own. Of course your personal or institutional resources will dictate this.

To improve your research and make transcription easier it is helpful to use quality equipment. There are many different contemporary recording devices available with much of this being digital. This means that many of the newer devices have large storage capacity and can be directly transferred onto your computer (Paulus et al., 2014). The microphone on your device will be crucial as this is what picks up the sound. Many devices have a built in microphone but this may not be adequate for research and you may want to invest in an external microphone to improve the quality of the audio. Some microphones have noise cancelling which can filter out extraneous background noises and can be very useful for research.

> When choosing a recording device remember to consider the battery life and whether it has a mains electric option.

Some mobile 'smart' phones have recording devices on them and this can be sufficient for a small project. Some even have video capability (Paulus et al., 2014). If you decide to use your smart phone as your recording device you will need to think about the storage capacity, the battery life and the protection of the data. It is helpful to remember that any digital file, whether stored on a computer, phone or other device should be encrypted to protect the participants. Not all devices have encryption software but it can be added to many. If it cannot be used on your device then make sure you transfer the files from the device to the computer where they can be password protected as soon as possible and delete the original.

> Do not delete the original file until you have checked the copy all the way through to make sure that it has copied properly.

Using video for mental health research

You may have noticed that there is rising pressure in health and mental health to produce quality evidence and this pressure has led to an increased use of recordings. The use of video in research allows clinical professionals to reflect upon their work which is made possible through the partnerships between researchers and practitioners (Carroll et al., 2008). This can be especially helpful in mental health research whereby professionals may use the research recordings to reflect on their relationships with clients as well as important aspects of their practice.

 Recruiting participants to studies that intend to video or audio record them can be a significant challenge for researchers (Themmessl-Huber et al., 2008).

Whether you plan to record the naturally occurring intervention, such as the therapy consultation/school classroom, or whether you plan to interview the children about their condition, the presence of a recording device may present an additional challenge in terms of how open or comfortable the child is to talk about his/her experiences. For effective research it is helpful to have the recording, but with sensitive topics this may create some discomfort. Research indicates that when patients report sensitive complaints (such as mental health difficulties) they are less likely to consent to participate in research, particularly young people who might be embarrassed by their condition (Themmessl-Huber et al., 2008).

Nonetheless using video to record research has increased and by using video you can engage professionals in taking a reflexive position in their work. If you do opt for recording naturally occurring mental health interactions then using video will allow you to observe professional action and focus on how professionals interact with their clients (Perakyla, 2006).

 If you do choose to use video-recordings remember that the children's consent is iterative. In other words consent should be dealt with as an on-going research concern (O'Reilly et al., 2011).

Using video with children in research

Most children in contemporary Western societies are growing up with technology. As we illustrated in Chapter 11, children are generally familiar with technology such as televisions, computers and digital equipment. From an early age children are typically photographed and often filmed by parents or other family members for personal reasons. If you choose to video children for your research this familiarity with equipment can be helpful, but do not assume that just because children are familiar with being recorded they are comfortable with it. Remember that the research context is quite different to their usual environment and that the issue of mental health is not necessarily an area they are comfortable to be recorded discussing. Recording children for research may make them nervous although children often report not feeling uncomfortable in the presence of a video camera (Grant & Luxford, 2009). There are certain steps you can take to help children feel more at ease and Bottorff (1994) cites four main ways:

1. Make sure you tell your participants the rationale for why you are using video to record them as this will help them understand the reasons behind your decisions.
2. Provide your participants with details about the data collection and how the process will unfold.
3. Assure your participants that the data will be protected and that their information will remain confidential.
4. Be careful where you place the camera so that it is not obtrusive and that participants are not constantly reminded of its presence.

There are challenges you may face if you video record children in the context of mental health and it is important you take steps to reduce these. This is important for the quality of your research and for the protection of your child participants. To help you we present the emotional challenges with some suggested solutions in Table 12.3 and the practical ones in Table 12.4.

Although it can be challenging to use video with children it is a useful way of gaining rich and detailed data. Children do talk about sensitive issues in front of a camera and notably are able to make the distinction

Table 12.3   Emotional challenges of using video with children

Challenge	Potential solution
Children may become uncomfortable or embarrassed during the recording.	It is essential that you assure the children that they can ask for the recording to stop at any time or ask for a break (Bottorff, 1994; O'Reilly et al., 2011).
The recording equipment may make the child anxious (Blaxter et al., 2001).	Some children may be more nervous than others and this may relate to the nature of their mental health difficulty, their age or other factors. Try to put the children at ease and build rapport with them, allow them to look at the equipment and see how it works and explain in detail what will happen and when. Furthermore think about where you position the cameras and/or microphones.
Children may worry about what they look like on camera in terms of their clothing, weight or other things that matter to them (Grant & Luxford, 2009).	It will be important that you give the children and their parents advanced warning that they will be on video so that they may take additional care over their appearance. Choosing clothes may create anxiety, so a school uniform may be helpful, or a dress code. Some reassurance may be helpful and consulting parents about potential anxieties in advance may also help you overcome any issues.

Table 12.4   Practical challenges of using video with children

Challenge	Potential solution
The use of video may further complicate existing power relations (Sparrman, 2005).	If time permits and you feel the child can be trusted to operate expensive equipment safely, you could allow them to record you first, letting them press buttons and review what they have recorded to give them some power over the situation. Make sure that they are aware that they can request a break and can ask for the camera to be stopped at any time. If the video recorder has a remote control it is useful to place this between you and give the child permission to press the stop button if they feel they want to.
Capturing children in noisy environments is difficult and the camera may not pick up everything that is wanted (Plowman & Stephen, 2008)	If you are recording children in a noisy environment such as the school classroom then you may miss important verbal information and these things cannot be recaptured if missed. This is something you need to consider at the planning stage of your research. If the verbal material is less important this may be acceptable, another environment may be preferable otherwise.
The presence of the video camera has the potential to unduly influence the behaviour of the participants.	Speer and Hutchby (2003) note, however, that this is not necessarily true or problematic and does not necessarily make the behaviour 'unnatural'. Furthermore research indicates that children tend to become acclimatised to the presence of the camera and forget about it (Bottorff, 1994).

between the social person (you) and the object (camera) (Sparrman, 2005). It is clear you need to take some responsibility for explaining why you are using a video camera, give them plenty of advance warning and allow them to be actively involved in the recording.

 A recording can never record the completeness of interaction and can be limited by issues of technical quality, background noise, zoom and where it is placed (Hamo et al., 2004).

Transcription

The next logical step from recording your data is to transcribe it (Lapadat, 2000). This is not as simple as it may sound. Transcription used to be viewed as technical and was viewed as unproblematic (Lapadat & Lindsay, 1999) but this myth was challenged by Ochs (1979) who argued that transcripts are actually selective and reflect the goals of the study. The vast literature now illustrates how transcription is understood as theoretical, selective, representational and interpretive with many different views of transcription available (Davidson, 2009).

> ## Example
>
> In linguistic anthropology transcription is seen as a cultural activity (Duranti, 2007).

> ## Example
>
> In sociolinguistics transcription is seen as a political act (Green et al., 1997).

> ## Example
>
> In conversation analysis transcription is seen as a situated practice (Mondada, 2007).

There are other traditions of transcription which view it in different ways but hopefully you can see there are important theoretical differences regarding the value and purpose of transcription. Transcription involves making selective decisions about the details of how what is said is included in the transcript and what details of prosody or intonation, for example, may be reasonable to leave out. It relies on the cultural knowledge and skills of the transcriptionist to interpret and represent what is going on in the audio/visual data (Hammersley, 2010).

> Remember that the transcript is not your data, but is a secondary product of representation to facilitate analysis (Mondada, 2007).

There are many important decisions to make before you begin transcribing and Hammersley (2010) outlines nine of the most important:

1. Decide how much of the recording to transcribe – the whole recording or just segments you want to analyse.
2. Decide how to represent your recorded talk as there is much variation of opinion amongst experts regarding how detailed a transcript you need.
3. Consider how to indicate who is speaking and who is being addressed in the talk.

4. Decide how much detail to include regarding audible non-words. This includes actions such as coughing, sneezing, laughing, crying and so forth.
5. Decide whether to represent the pauses in talk and whether to time them or simply differentiate short from long pauses.
6. Make decisions whether to include relevant gestures and fine motor movements.
7. Think about the layout of the text and how you represent overlapping or interruptive talk.
8. Make decisions regarding how to represent your participants as there is some contention about using numbers or pseudonyms.
9. When using a particular extract from the overall transcript you will need to decide where to start and end that extract and whether to include the interviewer's question (if there is one).

Making these decisions will not be easy and will rest on the theoretical assumptions of your work, the purpose of your research and your research questions. Probably one of the most important decisions you will need to make is the amount of detail to transcribe. You need to decide whether you are going to transcribe as the person speaks, with its incorrect pronunciation, grammar and accents, whether you are going to include mono/bi-syllabic sounds such as 'hum', 'okay' and 'uhuh', whether you are going to include actions such as sneezing and crying and other such details.

Transcription detail tends to be on a spectrum, from minimal verbatim transcription through to a highly detailed precise transcription. The decision rests on the amount of analytic relevance. For example in conversation the transcript aims to preserve the relevant vocal, verbal and multimodal details of the interactional event (Jefferson, 2004). This is because no detail in the interaction can be dismissed as irrelevant (Hepburn & Bolden, 2013). One of the factors which may influence your decision is the amount of time it takes to produce the transcript:

Example

A 30-minute interview can take 2–6 hours of transcription time depending on the level of detail (Lucas, 2010).

Example

To include the level of detail for a transcription for conversation analysis can take 1 hour for every 1 minute of tape (Roberts & Robinson, 2004) and can take even longer for video data.

Consider how different transcripts look. To help you visualise how data can be transcribed in different ways we take an extract of data from one of our papers (Parker & O'Reilly, 2012) and represent it in three different ways:

Example 1   Verbatim

FT: Mandy I'm going to talk to you because
Mum: Yeah
FT: you have been sat very patiently listening to
Mum: It's alright
FT: what two what two men have been saying almost about you and almost like we're gossiping gossiping in front of you.

If you have had a look at the actual paper you will see that this is not how the transcript is represented. What we have done here is represent the transcript verbatim. This means that we have illustrated what was said and corrected some of the grammar. This version has very little detail but does show the words that were spoken.

Example 2   Some details

FT: <u>Mandy</u>, I'm gonna talk to you cuz
Mum: Yeah
FT: you've been sat <u>very</u> patiently listening to
Mum: It's <u>al</u>right
FT: what two what two <u>men</u> <u>ha</u>ve been saying ((short pause)) erm almost about you and <u>al</u>most like we're <u>go</u>ssiping
Mum: ((mother laughs))
FT: gossiping in <u>fr</u>ont of you erm

In this example some of the details have been transcribed to give the reader some sense of how the words were spoken and other features such as laughter, which may be important in analysis later. Where words are emphasised the word is underlined in the transcript to show that this emphasis occurred. Short and long pauses are differentiated and mono/bi-syllabic words (e.g. 'erm') are included.

> ## Example 3   Very detailed (using Jefferson transcription systems)
>
> FT: <u>Man</u>dy, [I'm gonna talk t' you cuz =
> Mum: [↑Yeah
> FT: = you've be:en sat <u>ve</u>ry <u>pa</u>tiently lis[tenin' t' =
> Mum: [It's <u>a</u>lright
> FT: = what t' what t- two <u>men</u> 'ave be:en sayin' (0.4) e::rm almost
>   <about you> and <u>al</u>most like we're <u>go</u>ssipin'
> Mum: Heh heh heh
> FT: gossipin' in <u>fr</u>ont of you e::rm

In this example a very high level of detail is provided. Jefferson transcription notation (Jefferson, 2004) provides a set of symbols to represent certain ways in which talk is uttered. If you are unfamiliar with these conventions then some of the symbols can appear confusing and it can make the transcript more difficult to read. However, it is a more accurate way of representing the talk as it indicates where overlapping speech occurs, times the pauses in conversation, illustrates emphasis and changes in pace and intonation, does not correct grammar and includes social actions such as laughter.

 Whatever decisions you make require a rationale and are not merely a technical step of representing the talk (Skukauskaite, 2012).

 Activity   Table of pros and cons

Looking at the three extracts, try to produce a table of benefits and limitations of each of the styles of representation. Which version do you think is most suitable for your research based on this?

Transcribing children's talk

There are some additional transcription considerations when transcribing children's talk. Children speak differently to adults and their language is developing. The age group of the children will make a difference to how sophisticated their language and vocabulary are, but pronunciation and grammar may be less well developed so you will need to consider how to represent this in your transcripts.

Transcribing children's language is challenging (Davidson, 2009) as children's language involves constant and sudden shifts in role, voice and key (Hamo et al., 2004). There are occasions where people will use noises rather than speaking in words and there may be no current orthodox transcription notation for these sounds, but they have been referred to as 'active noising' (O'Reilly, 2005a). Children with certain mental health difficulties may also have problems in communication, may stutter or have problems completing sentences. This can make it very difficult to represent through a transcript.

The ways in which researchers represent children's talk in transcripts can emphasise the adult speakers' turns, meaning that the issue of power and the transcription layout and technique can inadvertently privilege adult's language over children's (Ochs, 1979). It is important to find ways of representing children's contributions in your transcript that challenge these cultural assumptions. This may necessitate being open to the information that you need being presented in a different form than you were expecting. For example, in interactions where adults and children are present, children's contributions may be interpreted as interruptions or distractions if they do not appear to be closely related to the question posed or current topic of conversation as initiated by the adult participants (O'Reilly, 2006).

However, in a similar way to our discussion about children giving 'assent' to participation in your research project rather than 'consent' (Chapter 4), children may express or indicate either their discomfort with or interest in the topic in different ways to adults. Either due to developmental maturation or the influence of a mental health difficulty, children often communicate in a less verbally articulate way than adults. Nevertheless, by 'tuning in' to their communication style or representational schema, it can be possible to hear what children are expressing in their own representational way. This may be through non-verbal ways (such as getting up and moving around, sighing, looking away, shrugging, belching, covering the face or putting up a hood), or by interjecting topic shifts (such as asking questions that seem unrelated, complaining, talking about something else, shouting). In your transcript, where non-verbal information is not included, you may arrive at your analysis stage and potentially misrepresent the child's contribution. By choosing not to include these features, your transcript may look like the child has not responded to a question/comment, but if you go back to your original data you may see that the child has communicated a response in a different way through gesture or audible but non-word utterances.

 Remember that the audio/video material is your data. The representation as a transcript will be a version of that (just as a painting is a version of a landscape).

Issues of translating for different languages

An increasing amount of research is now performed in languages other than English (Nikander, 2008). You may find you are undertaking your data collection in your native language and then translating the transcription into English, or another language. Often international conferences and journals require the presentation of the data in English. Despite this becoming much more common the issue of translation has been less well examined and neither have the power relations that are embedded in translation (Wong & Poon, 2010).

The limited literature and debate about the issues of translation reflects the taken-for-granted assumption that transcription is an objective neutral process and in which the translator is a mere technician in producing the text (Wong & Poon, 2010). However, as we illustrated earlier, transcription is not a neutral process and therefore neither is translation. Translating data is not simply a question of adopting or following a transcription technique but involves a range of practical and ideological questions related to the level of detail and the way in which words are physically presented (Nikander, 2008).

There are different ways of presenting transcripts in order that the native language is maintained. Nikander (2008) recommends choosing one of two principal ways:

1. First present the data in three lines, the original native language, the exact literal word-by-word translation and your 'tidied up' translation.
2. Second you can present parallel transcription with one language in the left column and the other language in the right.

For our first example we provide some data that was collected in Russian and translated into English. In the second example we provide data that was collected in English and translated into Greek. We show both forms of translation to illustrate the problems of representation. We thank Nadzeya Svirydzenka for the Russian and Panos Vostanis for the Greek.

Example 1   Translating from Russian to English

Russian: Что нужно изменить, чтобы сделать специализированную психиатрическую помощь более современной и результативной?

Literal: What necessary change, to make specialised mental health care more modern and efficient?

Translation: What do we need to change to make the specialised psychiatric help more contemporary and efficient?

(Continued)

(Continued)

Russian: Приоритетом реформирования является перерасп ределение ресурсов в пользу тех форм, эффекти вность которых не вызывает сомнений.

Literal: Priority reforming is distribution resources in benefit those forms, effectiveness which doesn't cause doubt.

Translation: Priority in the reform should be given to the redistribution of resources in favour of forms with guaranteed effectiveness.

Russian: Но прежде всего должно быть учтено мнение р одителей и детей, которые будут получать пси хиатрические услуги.

Literal: But before all must be taken opinion parents and children, which will receive psychiatric services.

Translation: However, above all, we should take into account the opinion of parents and children who will be receiving the mental health services.

Example 2 Translating from English to Greek

FT:	Mandy, I'm gonna talk to you cuz	Θεραπευτης Οικογενειας: Μαντυ, θα σου μιλησω, γιατι ετσι
Mum:	Yeah	Μαμα: Ναι
FT:	you've been sat very patiently	Θεραπευτης Οικογενειας: Περιμενες με πολλη υπομονη

Problematically, two languages do not map onto one another directly and some of the context can be lost in translation. For example, when translating the English data for a Greek audience some of the words are not fully translatable and alternatives need to be used. The mother in English says 'yeah', which is a slang term for yes, but as there is no slang term in Greek, the translation uses the word 'yes' – 'Ναι'. 'Sat patiently' does not translate to Greek easily and an alternative of 'waited patiently' is used instead. It is important to note that these small issues can matter to analysis and should be kept in mind during transcription.

Whichever form of representation you choose it is important you include the native language. If your child participants spoke in another language then their original talk must be represented that way in the transcript. By having the original language represented then international researchers are able to make judgements about your data and your conclusions (Nikander, 2008).

Financial aspects of transcription

You may prefer to employ a professional transcriptionist and this is fairly common (Tilley, 2003). If you have a budget then paying someone else to do the verbatim transcript can save time. Just because the transcriptionist provides you with the verbatim transcript does not mean that you can leave it as a complete task, however. You will need to listen to your data and go through each transcript, checking accuracy and adding in your desired level of detail. You will need to check that the transcriptionist has not 'tidied up' your data, that there are no errors or altered words and that the final transcript is anonymous and free from identifying details (Tilley & Powick, 2002).

It is important that you provide the transcriptionist with direction. It is helpful to spend some time talking to the transcriptionist regarding what you want with a time-frame. You will need to discuss how you want the data represented on the page, the layout of the text, the font you want and so forth.

 If you fail to give the transcriptionist an adequate level of direction they are likely to make their own decisions regarding how to represent the participants in the text (Tilley & Powick, 2002).

While paying someone to do this task is common there are arguments regarding the impact that this has on the quality of your work. Some argue that researchers should transcribe their own data as the process of transcription is important for analysis and in itself can yield important insights (Lapadat & Lindsay, 1999). This does have to be balanced against the advanced clerical skills that are needed to undertake accurate transcription in a timely manner (Halcomb & Davidson, 2006).

Protecting the transcriptionist

If you do pay someone to transcribe then remember you have some responsibility for their welfare. When the individual is transcribing they must repeatedly listen to your data and in this way disturbing events can become embedded into the consciousness of the transcriptionist (Gregory et al., 1997). As your research is on child mental health it is possible that this sensitive subject may lead to some distressing stories being told or upsetting emotions displayed by participants. It may be quite difficult for transcriptionists to detach from hearing stories of child abuse, self-harm or depression, for example.

The impact of listening to these traumatic stories can lead to vicarious traumatisation (Etherington, 2007) which is a process whereby the experience of empathically engaging with others' trauma narratives and experiences negatively affects the hearer (Pearlman & Saakvitne, 1995). Some of the emotional experiences of the children and their families displayed in your data may resonate with the transcriptionist and this can also create an emotional response. This is an important issue to consider when choosing a transcriptionist and when setting up the terms of your contract. It may be necessary for the transcriptionist him/herself to be offered some emotional support to manage the potential impact on them (Gregory et al., 1997). It is therefore important that you have regular contact with the transcriptionist, work as part of a team and warn them before they commit to the work if you believe that any of the content could be potentially distressing (Lalor et al., 2006; Parker & O'Reilly, 2013).

Summary

This chapter has introduced you to two important aspects of qualitative research, recording and transcription. First we illustrated some challenges related to recording your data. We contrasted audio with video and considered some of the practical and ethical challenges associated with each. We concluded that part of the chapter by considering the issues pertinent to using recording with children and more specifically regarding mental health research. The second part of the chapter focused on issues related to transcribing. We considered different forms of transcription and presented some of the debates that exist. The chapter concluded by considering some of the sensitivities invoked by transcribing sensitive topics and provided a caution to think about protecting the emotional well-being of the transcriptionist.

Key messages

- Digital technology has led to a greater reliance on audio and video recordings in qualitative research as this provides more detail than field notes.
- Audio and video recordings have practical and ethical challenges that need to be considered at the planning stages.

- Transcription is an active process and is underpinned by theoretical assumptions.
- It is important that researchers consider the emotional impact of the transcription process.

Further reading

Nikander, P. (2008). Working with transcripts and translated data. *Qualitative Research in Psychology*, 5, 225–231.

O'Reilly, M., Parker, N. & Hutchby, I. (2011). Ongoing processes of managing consent: The empirical ethics of using video-recording in clinical practice and research. *Clinical Ethics*, 6, 179–185.

Parker, N. & O'Reilly, M. (2012). 'Gossiping' as a social action in family therapy: The pseudo-absence and pseudo-presence of children. *Discourse Studies*, 14(4), 1–19.

PART FOUR
ANALYSIS AND WRITING-UP

CHAPTER 13

DATA ANALYSIS

Learning outcomes

- Appreciate that there are many different qualitative analytic approaches.
- Differentiate between the different analytic approaches.
- Identify the practical steps in undertaking qualitative analysis.
- Determine the appropriateness of computer software in aiding coding.

Introduction

This chapter is not intended to be a comprehensive guide to each analytic method. It is, however, important that you make an informed choice regarding your approach regarding which is most congruent with your theoretical framework and research question. This chapter serves as an introduction to the main analytic approaches but it will be necessary to use the information to select more specialised texts in that area. We provide you with some important practical information about each of the approaches so that you will have a basic understanding to enable an informed decision. With each approach we provide you with some step-by-step guidance relating to how to use the analytic method, reminding you that the process is rarely linear and we clarify some of the benefits and limitations of each method.

Thematic analysis

Thematic analysis is commonly used in qualitative research and if you are completely new to qualitative work it is a good way to develop your skills. Thematic analysis is epistemologically flexible, which means that it is compatible with many of the theoretical positions available. Thematic analysis is a helpful method to organise your data as it enables you to identify, analyse and report patterns within your data (Braun & Clarke, 2006). Using thematic analysis you will be able to make simple interpretations by describing what is going on within the data (Boyatzis, 1998).

 Thematic analysis is more than just themes emerging from the data (Braun & Clarke, 2006).

Thematic analysis can be used on most types of qualitative child data including interviews, focus groups, qualitative questionnaires, documents and video-taped materials (Joffe & Yardley, 2004). To start you need to code all of your data and then break it down into themes. A theme is something that captures something important in the data and will reflect what your research question is seeking to address (Braun & Clarke, 2006).

 To do thematic analysis effectively you will need to go through your actual data (that is the tapes/digital files) repeatedly alongside the transcripts to familiarise yourself with the content.

There is a clearly defined process to undertaking thematic analysis and we provide you with a practical step-by-step guide in Figure 13.1. We also recommend that you read Braun and Clarke, 2006.

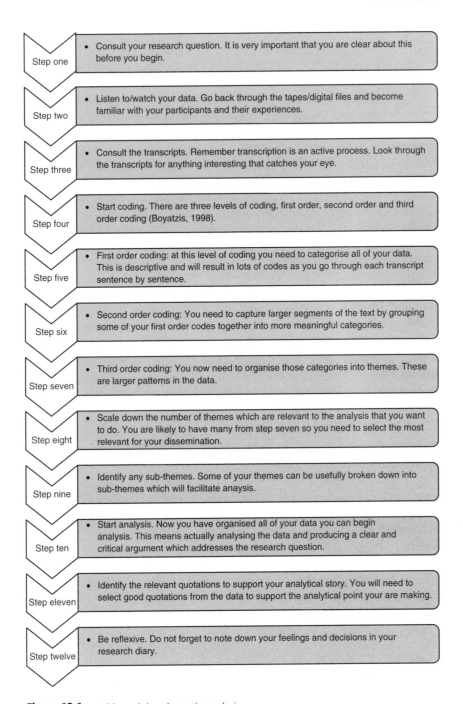

Step one • Consult your research question. It is very important that you are clear about this before you begin.

Step two • Listen to/watch your data. Go back through the tapes/digital files and become familiar with your participants and their experiences.

Step three • Consult the transcripts. Remember transcription is an active process. Look through the transcripts for anything interesting that catches your eye.

Step four • Start coding. There are three levels of coding, first order, second order and third order coding (Boyatzis, 1998).

Step five • First order coding: at this level of coding you need to categorise all of your data. This is descriptive and will result in lots of codes as you go through each transcript sentence by sentence.

Step six • Second order coding: You need to capture larger segments of the text by grouping some of your first order codes together into more meaningful categories.

Step seven • Third order coding: You now need to organise those categories into themes. These are larger patterns in the data.

Step eight • Scale down the number of themes which are relevant to the analysis that you want to do. You are likely to have many from step seven so you need to select the most relevant for your dissemination.

Step nine • Identify any sub-themes. Some of your themes can be usefully broken down into sub-themes which will facilitate anaysis.

Step ten • Start analysis. Now you have organised all of your data you can begin analysis. This means actually analysing the data and producing a clear and critical argument which addresses the research question.

Step eleven • Identify the relevant quotations to support your analytical story. You will need to select good quotations from the data to support the analytical point your are making.

Step twelve • Be reflexive. Do not forget to note down your feelings and decisions in your research diary.

Figure 13.1 Guide to doing thematic analysis

The process of thematic analysis is straightforward, but not easy to do well. Nonetheless using thematic analysis to explore children's mental health experiences can be beneficial as there are a number of advantages to this approach:

- It is a flexible method which is not tied to a particular theoretical position.
- All aspects of the children's narratives can be given full attention.
- It can describe data in a way that is accessible to a range of different child mental health audiences, including the children themselves.
- It can usefully highlight similarities and differences between children.
- You may be able to use your findings to inform policy development.

As with many methods there are some limitations of using thematic analysis to explore child mental health and you will need to consider how these may be overcome in practice:

- With large volumes of data it can be quite difficult for you to decide what to focus on.
- Thematic analysis is a descriptive method and therefore you will not be able to go beyond description.

A   Activity   Thematic analysis

With any analytic method it is important to look at the work of others. We recommend that you take some time now to look at some child mental health papers that have used thematic analysis. Do a Google Scholar search or look at this one:

O'Reilly, M., Cook, L. & Karim, K. (2012). Complementary or controversial care? The opinions of professionals on complementary and alternative interventions for Autistic Spectrum Disorder. *Clinical Child Psychology and Psychiatry, 17*(4), 602–615.

Grounded theory

The purpose of grounded theory is to generate theory. Originally, grounded theory was developed by Glaser and Strauss. In the grounded theory method you progressively move through your data to identify and integrate categories to finally produce a theory. To achieve this you will need to code your data simultaneously as you continue your data collection. In the early stages of analysis coding is largely descriptive as labels are assigned to discrete chunks of data (Willig, 2001). You will need to engage in constant comparative analysis to do this method properly and this means that you will have to go back and forth between data to look at the similarities and differences between emerging categories (Charmaz, 2006).

In grounded theory you continue recruiting participants and collecting data until you reach theoretical saturation. This is not the same as

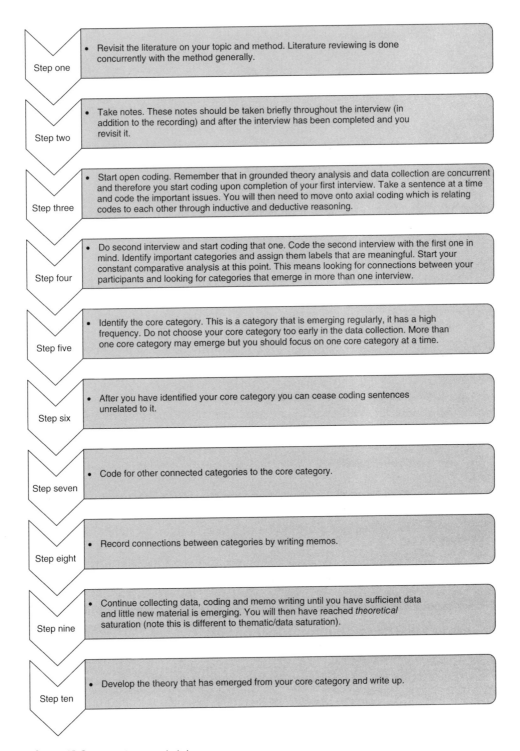

Figure 13.2 Steps in grounded theory

thematic/data saturation. Data saturation means that you stop recruiting when participants are starting to repeat what others have said so that nothing new is emerging. This means that you can start analysis. In grounded theory, you analyse and collect data simultaneously so you are identifying categories in the data and comparing them. When no new categories can be identified in the data you can stop collecting data because theoretical saturation has been reached.

There is a clearly defined process to undertaking grounded theory and we provide you with a practical step-by-step guide in Figure 13.2. We also recommend that you read Charmaz, 2005 and 2006.

Undertaking grounded theory is more complex than thematic analysis and it is advisable that you undertake training first. It is important you have a good understanding of the benefits and limitations of using this method and there are some clear advantages:

- This method will allow you to become immersed in the child data.
- Analysis is systematic and there is a clear method to follow.
- Analysis starts early so interesting issues raised by the children can be explored further.
- The data can be used as evidence for any claims that you may make.
- The method produces data which is rich in detail.

While this may seem appealing you need to be careful to consider the limitations of this method in producing a rationale for its use in your research:

- Coding for grounded theory may feel overwhelming, particularly if you are new to it.
- The high level of detail can make it difficult to project the more holistic picture.
- Grounded theory tends to produce lower level theory, rather than sophisticated theory.
- Open coding is very time-consuming, do not underestimate this.
- It is questionable whether one core category really can explain it all.

Interpretative phenomenological analysis

There are at least two distinct groups of phenomenological psychologists, descriptive and interpretative. Descriptive phenomenology is related to the work of Husserl and seeks to describe the essential structure of an experience, whereas the interpretative tradition is more interested in understanding the life-world, in terms of understanding individuals' experiences.

Interpretative phenomenological analysis, henceforth IPA, has grown in popularity recently and heavily utilises four key concepts:

1. Temporality – the experience of time.
2. Spatiality – the experience of space.
3. Intersubjectivity – the experiences of relationships with others and social groups.
4. Embodiment – the experience and connection to one's own body.

IPA aims to explore in depth the personal lived experiences of children to appreciate how they make sense of their lives. IPA is hermeneutic in the sense that the participant is trying to make sense of their personal and social world and the researcher is trying to make sense of the participant trying to make sense of their personal and social world (Smith, 2004). Smith (2004) notes, that there are three central characteristics of IPA:

1. It is idiographic.
2. It is inductive.
3. It is interrogative.

It is idiographic in that it starts with a detailed examination of one case before moving on, it is inductive in that researchers employ techniques that are flexible and it is interrogative in that it shares some constructs and concepts with mainstream psychology.

There is a clearly defined process to undertaking IPA and we provide you with a practical step-by-step guide in Figure 13.3. We also recommend that you read Smith, 2004.

By this point you should be clear that it is necessary to acknowledge and account for the benefits and limitations of your analytic method. IPA has some important advantages that may help you determine whether it is an appropriate approach for you:

- It provides you with a detailed and in-depth account of children's experiences and life-worlds.
- It only requires small sample sizes to achieve depth, so if you only have access to a small number of children or if you are looking at a rare condition this can be helpful.
- This method allows you to become involved in the children's lives.
- It provides you with a mechanism for exploring the experiences of children from their own point of view.
- The method allows for creativity and freedom (Willig, 2001).

This level of depth may seem attractive when exploring children's experiences and the small sample sizes can mean that it is a useful mode of

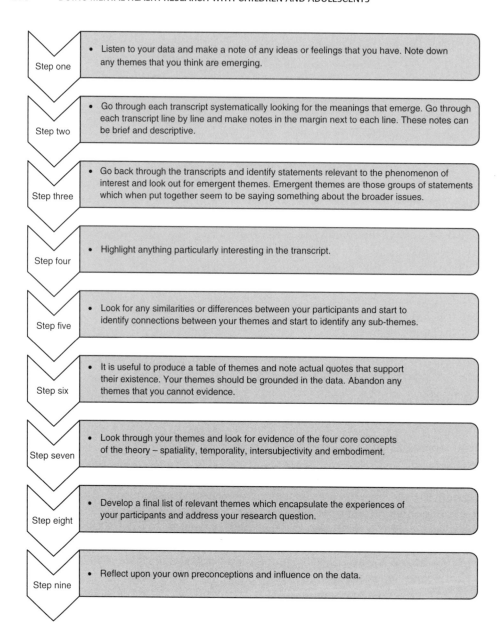

Figure 13.3 Steps involved in IPA

analysis. If you choose to undertake an IPA you do need to account for the limitations of this method:

- Analysis needs to be done in depth and therefore it can be very time consuming to conduct.
- It is possible that you may miss out important contextual details.

- IPA tends to use rather small sample sizes to achieve depth. While this may be an advantage, it can also be a source of criticism. It can make it difficult to enlighten in a broader context, limiting transferability.

Narrative analysis

Narrative analysis was pioneered by Labov in the early 1970s and focuses on the ways people use stories to interpret the world. This does not mean that they treat narratives as stories which offer facts about the world, rather they see narratives as social products which are produced in a particular context. Narrative analysis sees narratives as interpretative devices and it is through these that people represent themselves and their worlds to others (Riessman, 2005).

Narrative analysis is derived from narrative theory which argues that people produce accounts of themselves in the form of stories and that narrative is the key means through which a person's identity is produced (Riessman, 2005). Thus narrative analysis recognises the extent to which the stories people tell can provide insight into their experiences. By detecting the main narrative themes we can make sense of their lives (Thorne, 2000).

Narrative analysis is not easy to reduce to a number of practical steps and we therefore recommend that you undertake specialist training. There are some clear advantages to using narrative analysis for your work however, and it is helpful to consider these:

- Language is studied in context and you can control the context and its influence when studying your topic.
- Obtaining personal stories from children can provide you with rich and interesting data and you can collect these verbally or in writing.
- Narratives allow researchers to present children's experiences holistically rather than separating them out into categories.
- Analysing narratives allows you to reach experiences which the child may not be consciously aware of themselves.

As with any qualitative analytic technique there are some limitations of using narrative analysis and these should be balanced against the benefits:

- If you choose to obtain narratives in written form from children then this will depend on the cognitive and literacy abilities of the child.
- Narrative analysis is a time-consuming method of analysis and you will need to plan this into your time-frame.
- There are some ethical issues with this method as narratives are usually borne from friendships with the researcher and this rapport has potential to be misleading.

Discourse analysis

Discourse analysis (DA) has many variants underpinned by different theoretical assumptions and serves to answer different research questions. There are some differences between the different types of DA but there are some shared features:

- A focus on language.
- It acknowledges variability in people's accounts of things.
- It examines the broad regularities in the ways in which accounts are constructed.

The idea behind DA is that we 'do' things with language. We justify, question, invite and so forth using language and thus there is not an objective set of properties of events. In mental health we use language to construct illness and health. Therapy, counselling, psychology, education and psychiatry rely on language to understand children's conditions and therefore it makes some sense to choose an analytic method with a focus on language.

It is difficult to provide a single definition of DA as it is more of a set of principles and can be characterised as a commitment to studying discourse as talk and text in social practice. It is generally an umbrella term which encompasses a number of techniques for analysing discourse in practice. Over time a number of different types of DA have been developed and this can pose challenges for providing a full account of its methods. Morgan (2010) identifies six types of DA, but we introduce you to the more common types recommending you read further.

1. Discursive psychology (including the roots of the Potter and Wetherell form).
2. Critical discourse analysis.
3. Interactional sociolinguistics.
4. Bakhtinian discourse analysis.
5. Foucauldian discourse analysis.
6. Conversation analysis.

Traditional discourse analysis (Potter & Wetherell, 1987)

This form of DA is grounded in ethnomethodology and has a social constructionist framework. It uses three core concepts outlined in Table 13.1.

Discursive psychology

Discursive psychology (DP) reflects the key concerns of ethnomethodology and Wittgenstein's theory of language. This type of DA is heavily influenced

Table 13.1   The three core concepts

Concept	Description
Interpretive repertoire	Interpretive repertoires are the common sense (but contradictory) ways that people talk about the social world. They are common knowledge, the cultural ideas and explanations that everyone knows. Interpretive repertoires are used to build explanations, accounts and arguments (Potter & Wetherell, 1987).
Subject positions	This is the discursive process of locating the identity of others and oneself. In conversation we position others using adjectives or categories and position them in a certain way. We may position someone as a 'bad mother' which constructs the identity of that person in a particular way. This can then be accepted or rejected by others including the talked about person. We can position ourselves in the same way.
Ideological dilemmas	The concept of an ideological dilemma was developed by Billig et al. (1988) as a concept relating to the fragmented and contradictory nature of everyday common sense. Ideological dilemmas relate to common knowledge and cultural wisdom as being full of contradiction and many beliefs and expressed values are not fixed, rather they are lived ideologies. In other words they are ways of explaining and interpreting flexible rhetorical resources. So for example a modern father may have the ideological dilemma in a research interview of showing the interviewer that he is a good father who spends time with his children while managing the contradiction that he works 60 hours per week.

by conversation analysis and is concerned with how people report their mental states, arguing that mental state reports are social actions (Edwards & Potter, 1992). DP thus provides a general critique of cognitive theory and criticises the traditional methods used to study them. This is important for mental health research as this analytic approach argues that children's mental health difficulties are constituted in and reflected by language, rather than being fixed biological states.

DP grew from discourse analytic work that was interested in the way in which speakers draw on cognitive concepts such as memory or attention and make them relevant as a way of constructing fact (Wooffitt, 2005). It challenges the way we look at phenomena like identity and memory asserting that these are not entities in themselves but are constituted through language (Morgan, 2010). DP draws upon the principles of discourse and conversation analysis and key professionals are Derek Edwards, Alexa Hepburn, Elizabeth Stokoe and Jonathan Potter.

Critical discourse analysis

Critical discourse analysis grew out of linguistics, semiotics and discourse analysis. It is primarily concerned with theorising and researching social processes and social change. Critical DA focuses on political or social issues. This form has its roots in linguistics and has a primary interest in the role of discourse in the production of power within social structures. In other words it looks at how language manages to sustain and legitimise social inequality (Wooffitt, 2005). In the case of child mental health these analysts are interested in the power differentials between groups, such as children and therapists and those with mental health difficulties and those without. This type of DA would seek to investigate how the subordinate position of children with mental health difficulties is created through language and interaction.

Critical DA emerged from other forms of DA and conversation analysis but provides a critical edge by having a commitment to demystifying the dominant ideologies in society. The purpose of critical DA is to promote positive political social change (Morgan, 2010). Key professionals doing critical DA include Teun van Dijk, Norman Fairclough and Ruth Wodak.

Considering discourse analysis for your project

As there are many different types of DA you may find differentiating some of the subtle differences between them challenging. Your choice of which discourse approach to use will depend on the epistemological framework that you favour. Inevitably, if you choose to do DA for your project then you will need some specialised training. Learning the methods of DA requires time and patience. There are, however, some advantages of using this method:

- DA can be applied to any situation or subject where people talk or communicate.
- DA has potential to reveal the unspoken and unacknowledged aspects of human behaviour.
- DA is context specific.
- DA can generate important new insights.
- DA is a 'value free' method.
- DA is rigorous and systematic.
- Analysis is grounded in the data.

Although this list of advantages may be appealing it is important you acknowledge the limitations:

- DA cannot provide definite answers.
- Similarities and differences between concepts may cause confusion.
- There is a lack of step-by-step tools for doing DA.
- It is a complex method for novice researchers to employ.
- Some forms of DA are criticised for their political intentions.

Conversation analysis

Conversation analysis (CA) was developed in sociology. Harvey Sacks pioneered CA in the 1960s, growing from the work of Garfinkel who founded ethnomethodology. Garfinkel (1967) argued that people are able to under-stand and share sense of their interactions and circumstances and meaning-ful interactions are impossible without these shared understandings. Researchers use CA to explore mundane and institutional talk as a system-atic and organised phenomenon, giving attention to the detail in naturally occurring interaction (Wooffitt, 2005). Thus CA is known as exploring talk-in-interaction.

CA is used to examine the social organisation of activities produced through talk and looks at the sequential patterns of interaction (Hutchby & Wooffitt, 2008). This means that it looks at the turns at talk and identifies the ways that people's utterances occur in succession to form a pattern of interaction. Sacks et al. (1974) observe that CA focuses on the ways in which social realities are constituted through a person's talking-interaction. It is concerned with more than just talk. It is concerned with the organiza-tion of the meaningful conduct of people in society how they make sense of the world around them (Pomerantz & Fehr, 1997).

CA focuses on everyday talk in mundane or institutional settings and looks at how claims are made to appear neutral, stable and separate from the speaker (Potter, 1996). As with DA there is no simple step-by-step pro-cess to undertaking CA. It is a complex method and you will require spe-cialised training and expert supervision. There are, however, a number of advantages of using this technique for your research project:

- CA is a precise method which allows you to explore the detailed nuances of interaction.
- Analysis is grounded in the data.
- Audio and video data can be analysed in depth.
- It challenges the taken-for-granted view of language.
- It is a 'value free' method.
- It is rigorous and systematic.

Like other methods it is important that you consider the limitations of CA when constructing your methodological rationale:

- CA has a specialised transcription system (the Jefferson method) which is very time-consuming and resource intensive.
- You will need specialised training.
- The analytic process is open to potential misinterpretation.
- Obtaining naturally occurring data in child mental health is not easy.
- You will need a good quality recording and equipment can be expensive.

 You can only use conversation analysis on naturally occurring data.

Because of the epistemological framework of CA researchers using this method use naturally occurring data only. This can be quite challenging in the field of child mental health. You will need to carefully negotiate with institutional representatives, ethics committees, parents, children with mental health difficulties and possibly other family members to be able to audio or video record data (refer back to Chapter 10).

Final decisions

Now you have considered the different analytic methods and their respective benefits/limitations you should be able to make an informed decision regarding which is most appropriate for your research question. You should have considered the theory underpinning your research, the question being addressed and the type of data collection you are choosing to engage in. Consider the following activity to help you think about your choices.

Case example

Marco is a family therapist in a child mental health outpatient setting. His manager asked Marco to do a small-scale research project to explore children's views of their service. Marco has carried out 15 semi-structured interviews with children under the age of 16. Now he has his data he has got stuck and needs some advice on which analytic method to use. He comes to you because he does not know what to do with the data.

A   **Activity   Helping Marco**

What advice would you give to Marco?

You should note that Marco did not plan his research very well. He did not think about which perspective he wanted to utilise prior to data collection. Different analytic approaches determine the style and content of an interview and some approaches do not use interviews. Early in the chapter we illustrated that thematic analysis is epistemologically flexible so Marco might be able to consider this. This should remind you just how important it is to make your methodological decisions at the planning stage of your research.

NVivo

When you have made your decision regarding analytic method it is helpful to decide whether to use computer software to help you. Some types of qualitative analysis are well suited to the use of computer software to help you at the coding stages. Although there are different computer software packages available the most commonly used is NVivo, which can help you to manage large amounts of data.

> **!** Caution: Remember that NVivo will not do the analysis for you, rather it facilitates the coding process and helps you to organise your data (Bryman, 2008).

If you are going to use NVivo then it is useful to find training to learn the basics. To help you we provide you with a flow chart in Figure 13.4.

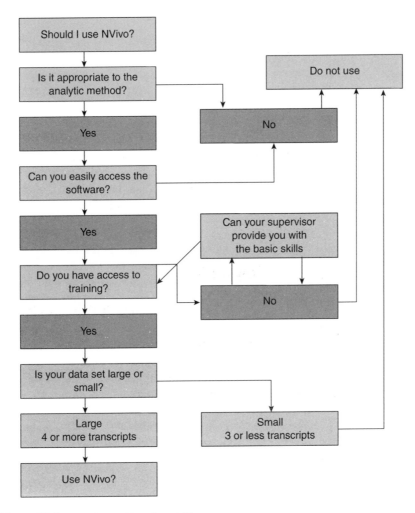

Figure 13.4   Decision-making about NVivo

It is useful to obtain a book from your library on NVivo to help you decide and to familiarise yourself with the terminology and process. It may feel quite daunting when you first encounter the programme as there are a number of terms used and commands operational.

To use NVivo it will be necessary to import your transcripts into the programme and then look at one transcript at a time. As you go through each transcript you can organise the chunks of information into labelled folders which you create as codes (in NVivo, these are Nodes). This means that the programme is helpful for any analytic method that requires you to code or categorise your data. Each of these codes/nodes can have a sub-folder attached to it. In practice this means that you will end up with a 'hierarchy tree' of folders which contain all of the codes you have assigned. These 'trees' allow you to add quotations from your transcripts into the folders (more than one if it fits more than one) and then print out just that single folder. This means that you can see all the quotations from your data that are assigned to a single code. You can also add memos to the project which can serve as useful reminders.

Summary

In this chapter we have introduced you to the main approaches of qualitative analysis. The form of analysis you choose to use for your research should be guided by your research question and epistemological position. In this chapter we have provided a simple overview of the main analytic approaches and given some practical guidance related to undertaking these methods. The chapter concluded with some discussion of computer software which may facilitate the coding process.

Key messages

- There are different methods of analysis which have different theoretical assumptions and processes.
- You will need to do some additional reading before you attempt to undertake your analysis.
- For some methods you may need specialised training.
- You may find it useful to use NVivo to facilitate your coding.

Further reading

Braun, V. & Clarke, V. (2006). Using thematic analysis in psychology. *Qualitative Research in Psychology, 3*, 77–101.

Charmaz, K. (2006). *Constructing grounded theory: Practical guide through qualitative analysis*. London: Sage.

Riessman, C. K. (2005). Narrative analysis. In N. Kelly, C. Horrocks, K. Milnes, B. Roberts & D. Robinson (eds), *Narrative, memory and everyday life* (pp. 1–7). Huddersfield: University Of Huddersfield.

Smith, J. A. (2004). Reflecting on the development of interpretative phenomenological analysis and its contribution to qualitative research in psychology. *Qualitative Research in Psychology, 1*, 39–54.

Wooffitt, R. (2005). *Conversation analysis and discourse analysis: A comparative and critical introduction.* London: Sage.

CHAPTER 14

REFLECTIVE PRACTICE TO REFLEXIVE RESEARCH

Learning outcomes

- Differentiate between clinical reflection and research reflexivity.
- Appreciate the reasons why research reflexivity is important.
- Practice research in a reflexive way.
- Assess the importance of the research supervisor.

Introduction

We open this chapter by introducing you to the important issue of reflexivity, outlining some similarities/differences with clinical reflection. We acknowledge that some of you will have experience of clinical reflection and while there are similarities, there are important differences. As the chapter unfolds you are introduced to some of the core concepts and we provide you with practical steps for being a reflexive child mental health researcher. The reasons why reflexivity is important are explained clearly and useful tips for engaging in this process effectively provided. Part of the reflexive process is to recognise and manage the emotional impact of working with sensitive topics. This is connected to the issue of research and clinical supervision and we consider ways in which you may use these two streams of supervision to your benefit.

Clinical reflection

Although 'reflection' is a complex concept that has no universally agreed definition (Johns & Freshwater, 1998), reflective practice is well established in clinical work and is the process of actively considering your clinical experiences. By reflecting upon what you do on a daily basis you can improve your skills by looking at what you do well and where your skills are limited. The concept of reflective practice was developed by Schön (1983) who argued there are two ways to engage in reflection:

1. Reflecting-on-action – reflection you do after the experience has finished.
2. Reflecting-in-action – when you are reflective during the experience.

Reflection in clinical work requires a process of self-involvement and self-reflection and enables you to become aware of the influence of ideological and societal assumptions, especially any moral or ethical beliefs which underpin your practice (Yip, 2006). It is clear that reflective practice is an important means for clinical learning (Boud et al., 1985) and it can help to enhance your personal and professional profile (Yip, 2006).

Research reflexivity

Research reflexivity has similarities with clinical reflection and you can certainly translate some of those skills to research. Nonetheless reflexivity is often confused with reflection, whereas in reality the two concepts can be thought of as on a continuum (Finlay, 2002). Finlay argues that the process of reflection is a distanced one where typically the thinking is done after the event has taken place, with reflexivity being a more immediate, continuing and dynamic self-awareness. This parallels Schön's 'reflection-in-action'.

Typically in research it refers to the process of examining how you have impacted upon and transformed the research process (Finlay, 2003). Basically it means that you make visible your own individuality and how this has impacted on your research (Gough, 2003). When you are engaging in the research process it is inevitable that you will influence the idea formation, data collection, selection of participants and interpretation (Finlay, 2002) so it is through communicated reflexivity that this becomes transparent. In research contexts there are two types of reflexivity, outlined by Willig (2001):

1. *Personal reflexivity* requires reflection on your values, attitudes, political commitments, experiences, beliefs and social identities, reflecting on the ways in which they may have impacted upon and shaped the research. Your views of children and childhood and of mental health will be instrumental here.
2. *Epistemological reflexivity* requires you to engage with your research question in terms of how that question is defined and limited and how the study design constructs the data. This type of reflexivity encourages you to reflect upon your theoretical assumptions and how these have shaped the findings.

This illustrates that one of the main differences between clinical reflection and reflexivity relates to the different styles of reflexivity and the different theoretical assumptions upon which it operates.

 When being reflexive it is important not to allow your own position to become unduly privileged and block out the voice of your participants (Finlay, 2002).

Why reflexivity is important

The literature on reflexivity indicates that there are three main reasons why it is important:

1. To embrace the influence researchers have on the research process.
2. To engage with the researcher's theoretical framework.
3. To attend to issues of quality.

Traditionally, quantitative research has sought to remove researcher bias from the process, with the influence of the researcher being viewed as problematic. In qualitative research however, the role of the researcher is considered to be enriching and informative; thus reflexivity is a mechanism through which researchers are able to make visible their individuality (Gough, 2003). It is considered important to embrace the influence you have had on this process and not to omit any aspect of yourself in that work.

Reflexivity is also considered important from a theoretical point of view. All qualitative research is underpinned by theory and there is diversity in regard to the epistemological positions of different qualitative researchers. It is important that you acknowledge this and reflect upon the assumptions that this has for your research and the findings as this will shape the process (Willig, 2001).

Finally, and perhaps most importantly, reflexivity is important for quality. We discussed issues of assessing quality in qualitative research in Chapter 2 and reflexivity is integral to this process. Integrity and trustworthiness are essential for judging the value of qualitative work and reflexivity is a process which makes transparent the research process (Finlay, 2003). Typically therefore the benefit of reflexive research practice relates to gaining a better understanding and explanation of your role in the research process to increase the transparency of the data and general integrity of the process (Nadin & Cassell, 2006).

_A_   **Activity   Reflexivity in your project**

In your diary write a list of the ways in which you think being a reflexive researcher might improve the quality of your work.

Professional case example   Interview with Dr Lester

Dr Jessica Lester (Indiana University) has written extensively on child mental health, particularly in the area of autism. We asked her some questions about using reflexivity to manage the quality of her research and deal with the sensitive data.

1 When undertaking your research with children diagnosed with autism, how did being reflexive help you stay emotionally healthy?

Throughout this work, being reflexive was a recursive practice – one sought with intentionality. From maintaining a reflexivity journal to finding ways to continually reflect on the research process, I recognised the value and importance of being reflexive. My own interpretations and sense of 'groundedness' were very much linked to the degree to which I practiced reflexivity. There were days when I questioned the nature of this type of work, particularly as I listened to the challenges of the parents of

(Continued)

(Continued)

children diagnosed with autism and the day-to-day struggles of the children. Quite often, I was challenged to think carefully about my own complicity in those systems that served to exclude the children. The children often shared (via drawings and/or through words) how they felt misunderstood. I was reminded often that I could easily be one of those who misunderstood them. As I engaged in reflexive practice, I considered my own role in society and that of others. Through reflexive practice, I worked to stay emotionally grounded and aware of my own subjectivities (at least in part) that shaped the research process.

2 Were there any challenges to watching sensitive video data?

One of the most significant challenges of viewing the video data was making sense of the nonverbal communication that was unfamiliar to me. I sought to make sense of the functional nature of the children's communication. Yet, at times, I found myself orienting to the children's communication from a deficit perspective, one which I intended to eschew. I found this to be a sensitive act, as asking children to allow me to videotape their therapy sessions suggested that I would view their therapeutic interactions with care and respect. I realised early on that viewing their tapes with care meant assuming that they were competent, regardless of the ways in which they chose to communicate. Thus, I was pushed to spend countless hours rethinking how I would go about analysing their interactions. This led me to spend time with the children's parents and therapists, asking them to 'teach' me to better understand the nature of their children's nonverbal communication. This allowed me to pursue an analysis that assumed competency and positioned the children as functional human beings.

How do you think your reflexive position helped you develop the quality of your research project?

Engaging in reflexive work pushed me to examine how my own subjectivities shaped the research process. Further, by recognising this reality, I was able to thoughtfully write myself into the research process, allowing others to recognise, critique, and respond to the nature of 'self' within the interpretative process. This served to increase the trustworthiness of my findings, as it created space for others to validate and make sense of my decision-making process. Additionally, my reflexive position was one that continually pushed me to rethink how

I was making sense of 'ethics' within the research process, which is foundational to any quality research study. Thus, in many ways, reflexivity grounded and centred my research practice.

Some useful references

Lester, J. N. (2012). A discourse analysis of parents' talk around their children's autism labels. *Disability Studies Quarterly, 32*(4), Art. 1.
Lester, J. N. & Paulus, T. M. (2012). Performative acts of autism. *Discourse & Society, 12*(3), 259 – 273.
There is more on her website: http://portal.education.indiana.edu/ProfilePlaceHolder/tabid/6210/Default.aspx?u=jnlester

How to be reflexive

Reflexivity is a process that starts from the beginning of your project through to dissemination. In order to write reflexively you need to ensure that you are actively engaged in reflexive thought at all stages and this is best demonstrated through your research diary. This is very important to enable you to demonstrate reflexivity and the use of your diary can also help you to develop a narrative about the context of your research, which will keep your work grounded (Nadin & Cassell, 2006). The collection of your reflective thoughts, memories, experiences and feelings will help you to write up your reflexivity during dissemination.

The way in which you write the reflexive component of your research in dissemination will depend on the purpose for which it is being written. Not all journals allow room for full reflexive prose and you will have to consider how much detail you include. A thesis/dissertation is, however, likely to require much more information. Consider these short excerpts from the PhD of one author (O'Reilly, 2005b) and a more current research project. Both of these examples are personal reflexivity (Willig, 2001) and consider the influence the researcher had on the research process.

Reflexivity

'It is possible that my own feelings about the inadequacy of help available to children with disabilities may have impacted on my choice of topics. Disability and child mental health as a broad topic within the

(Continued)

> *(Continued)*
>
> research is motivated by my curiosity about the lived experiences of disability. I lived with an autistic sibling through my childhood and have always been interested in whether other people experience it in a similar way. It is fair to assume therefore that without these preconceived ideas about disability and experience I may not have ever chosen to conduct this type of research at all and so its existence is dependent upon my frustration and curiosity.'

Please note that we are not setting this up as a perfect example. Indeed the author who wrote this has certainly learned much more about how to be reflexive since her PhD days! Nonetheless this example does give you a good impression of how reflexivity is constructed in practice. Using excerpts from the research diary it was noted that from its inception, the research was influenced by prior experiences of child mental health and indeed the motivation for undertaking the research rested upon personal experiences of living with autism.

Now consider this reflection from a more recent study by O'Reilly looking at autism through focus groups. This excerpt considers the author's feelings more directly in terms of how she felt conducting focus groups.

> ## Reflexivity
>
> 'Autistic Spectrum Disorder (ASD) is a lifelong neuro-developmental condition (Sharpe & Baker, 2007). While the research states this it is interesting to see how those who live with autism feel about it and with my brother's autism in the back of my mind I felt strongly about the issues raised. The member of the group with autism said he was happy with this fact but this is contrary to my brother who often becomes distressed, which made me feel tense. It is also contrary to research which shows that families of children with autism tend to be stressed (Bromley et al., 2004). This is however consistent with some of the recent voices such as Aspies. This tension made me tentatively challenge the claim.'

Using the diary to guide memory of the feelings invoked by interacting with the focus group, the author's emotions were acknowledged. It is important to recognise how you are feeling during the data collection process, not only to stay safe but also to think about how these emotions may influence the way you write up your research, what you may privilege in terms of analysis and the ways in which you develop your analytic points.

Using your supervisor

For your project you probably have a research supervisor, or at least a colleague/manager for support. If you are also a clinician then you probably have a clinical supervisor and there may be some overlap in the issues you choose to discuss with them. Your relationship with your research supervisor will be important and it is essential that you build this relationship early. You may/may not have a choice regarding who supervises your project but if you do then it is important to choose a supervisor with specialist knowledge of your topic and the methods you intend to use.

Good supervisors should give you clear and frequent indications regarding your performance (Abiddin et al., 2009). Remember that your supervisor is not there to 'spoon-feed' you, but to help you to foster independent learning (Thompson et al., 2005). Of course, bad supervisors exist and poor supervision can have considerable impact on you and the quality of your work (Abiddin et al., 2009). Magnuson et al. (2000) developed an interesting profile of poor supervision and we outline this in Table 14.1.

Table 14.1 Lousy research supervision (Magnuson et al., 2000)

Principle	Description
1 Unbalanced	The participants in their study cited the importance of balance in supervision and felt that an unbalanced supervisor was one who focused too much on the detail and failed to appreciate the broader picture.
2 Developmentally inappropriate	The participants in their study argued that some supervisors were developmentally inappropriate whereby the supervisor fails to recognise and respond to the changing needs of their research students.
3 Intolerant of differences	Participants identified that some research supervisors failed to allow their research students to be innovative and were impatient, rigid or inflexible in their supervisory approach.
4 Poor model of personal/professional attributes	Participants in this study identified that some supervisors failed to orient to the boundaries of research supervision and in some cases were intrusive and exploitative.
5 Untrained	Participants in the study recognised that some research supervisors had inadequate preparation or professional maturity for the role.
6 Professionally apathetic	Participants referred to the lousy supervisor as being the individual who lacked the commitment needed to perform the role adequately.

> Ultimately it is you who is responsible for your research project (Abiddin et al., 2009).

As noted it is you that has the final responsibility for your work. While it is helpful to have a good supervisor, you need to be a good student. O'Reilly et al. (2013) outline a number of practical hints for good supervision that you can do to facilitate the process:

- Remember your supervisor is busy and probably has several students so use your time wisely.
- Before supervision write down questions you want to ask; have a check-list of areas you want to cover so that you do not forget things.
- Email an agenda to your supervisor in advance of your supervision, so that you both know what is going to be discussed.
- Allow your supervisor sufficient time to give you feedback. You cannot submit something last thing on Friday and expect feedback on Monday.
- If you are doing your research as part of an educational project then your institution is likely to have a code of practice for supervision. Use this and understand it.
- Try to meet with your supervisor regularly.
- It is useful to have some notes from the supervision meetings as a reminder. Talk to your supervisor about how these are taken and by whom. An example is given in Figure 14.1.
- Remember your supervisor is not your counsellor and if you are having personal/emotional problems that are affecting your research then you may need to seek help elsewhere (clinical supervisors, if you have one, may be more appropriate here).

Obviously, Figure 14.1 contains reduced detail to illustrate an example. It would be expected that the key issues part would be more detailed and that the student uses their section for questions and to show achievements. Good supervision is a two-way process. This will be facilitated if both you and your supervisor are honest, work with integrity and ensure that data protection, intellectual property and copyright issues are addressed (Thompson et al., 2005). Effective communication will be essential on both sides and a good relationship should be built.

Summary

In this chapter we have focused on the importance of reflexivity in research, particularly in research in child mental health. We distinguished between clinical reflection and reflexivity while drawing your attention to some of

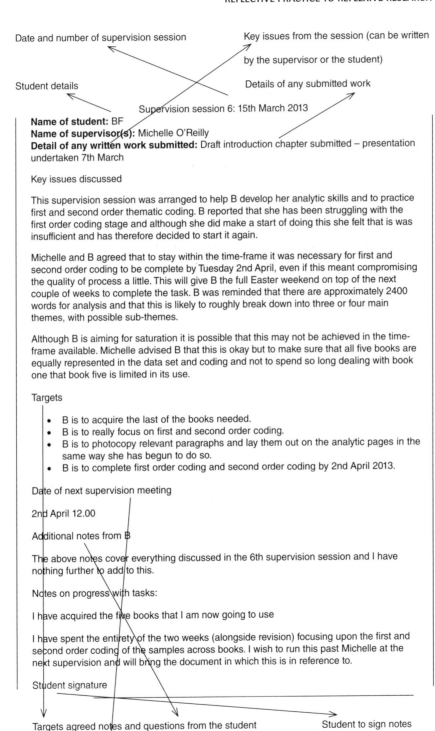

Date and number of supervision session

Key issues from the session (can be written by the supervisor or the student)

Student details

Details of any submitted work

Supervision session 6: 15th March 2013

Name of student: BF
Name of supervisor(s): Michelle O'Reilly
Detail of any written work submitted: Draft introduction chapter submitted – presentation undertaken 7th March

Key issues discussed

This supervision session was arranged to help B develop her analytic skills and to practice first and second order thematic coding. B reported that she has been struggling with the first order coding stage and although she did make a start of doing this she felt that is was insufficient and has therefore decided to start it again.

Michelle and B agreed that to stay within the time-frame it was necessary for first and second order coding to be complete by Tuesday 2nd April, even if this meant compromising the quality of process a little. This will give B the full Easter weekend on top of the next couple of weeks to complete the task. B was reminded that there are approximately 2400 words for analysis and that this is likely to roughly break down into three or four main themes, with possible sub-themes.

Although B is aiming for saturation it is possible that this may not be achieved in the time-frame available. Michelle advised B that this is okay but to make sure that all five books are equally represented in the data set and coding and not to spend so long dealing with book one that book five is limited in its use.

Targets

- B is to acquire the last of the books needed.
- B is to really focus on first and second order coding.
- B is to photocopy relevant paragraphs and lay them out on the analytic pages in the same way she has begun to do so.
- B is to complete first order coding and second order coding by 2nd April 2013.

Date of next supervision meeting

2nd April 12.00

Additional notes from B

The above notes cover everything discussed in the 6th supervision session and I have nothing further to add to this.

Notes on progress with tasks:

I have acquired the five books that I am now going to use

I have spent the entirety of the two weeks (alongside revision) focusing upon the first and second order coding of the samples across books. I wish to run this past Michelle at the next supervision and will bring the document in which this is in reference to.

Student signature

Targets agreed notes and questions from the student

Student to sign notes

The date of the next meeting

Figure 14.1   Supervision notes

the similarities between the two skills. Reflexivity is important in qualitative research and we have illuminated some of these reasons. This is facilitated by the engagement of a good research supervisor and we concluded this chapter with discussions regarding how to use the research supervision effectively.

Key messages

- Clinical reflection and research reflexivity are different but have many similarities.
- Reflexivity in qualitative research is important for quality, assessing the impact of the researcher and addressing theory.
- It is important to have a good, supportive supervisor to help you with your project.
- Ultimately the success of your project is down to you.

Further reading

Finlay, L. (2003). The reflexive journey: Mapping multiple routes. In L. Finlay & B. Gough (eds), *Reflexivity: A practical guide for researchers in health and social sciences* (pp. 3–20). Oxford: Blackwell Publishing.

Gough, B. (2003). Deconstructing reflexivity. In L. Finlay & B. Gough (eds), *Reflexivity: A practical guide for researchers in health and social sciences* (pp. 21–36). Oxford: Blackwell Publishing.

Magnuson, S., Wilcoxon, S.A. & Norem, K. (2000). A profile of lousy supervision: Experienced counselors' perspectives. *Counselor Education and Supervision, 39,* 189–202.

CHAPTER 15

DISSEMINATION

Learning outcomes

- Write a qualitative child mental health paper.
- Present at a conference.
- Know how to write a thesis or dissertation.
- Appreciate the ethical considerations of dissemination.
- Recognise the challenges of sharing findings with children.

Introduction

We open this chapter by considering two of the common ways to disseminate research; papers for journals and presenting at conferences. We discuss the strengths and limitations of each of these and provide practical guidance.

Some of you will be undertaking a project for an educational qualification and we provide some practical suggestions for writing a thesis/dissertation. In this chapter we consider the range of dissemination options including using the internet, preparing leaflets or using the media and give you some practical examples to help you. Additionally we recognise some of the challenges of dissemination generally and provide discussion regarding the ethics of dissemination. This is particularly pertinent in qualitative research and is important for child mental health. We conclude the chapter by discussing how to share your findings with your participants.

Why disseminate?

Broadly speaking dissemination is the delivery of knowledge and is designed to impact on practitioner behaviour/interaction and/or outcomes (Chorpita & Regan, 2009). In health (and in some other disciplines) there is a growing expectation that professionals present and publish their research (Cleary & Walter, 2004).

A   **Activity   Why disseminate?**

List three reasons why you think it is necessary to disseminate child mental health research.

There are many reasons why child mental health researchers/practitioners disseminate their findings. The reasons you could have considered include your responsibility to disseminate what you have found. You have an ethical obligation to share the findings of your research, as participants have given their time on the understanding that knowledge will be generated to inform practice and service provision. This is just as important if your study yielded negative findings so that others can learn from it. Disseminating your work means that knowledge is shared and therefore treatments, services, patient engagements and communication can potentially be improved. Additionally disseminating your work may contribute to policy decisions, particularly if your work is synthesised with other evidence to develop an important practice message. Dissemination can raise awareness of the issues that children and families face, rare conditions can be understood better, knowledge can be promoted and stigma may be reduced. Disseminating your research may also open communication with others interested in discussing future possibilities to build on your findings.

How to write a qualitative child mental health journal article

A common and desirable form of dissemination is journal articles. Publishing articles can help understand children's experiences, the process of therapeutic interventions, facilitate engagement and develop partnerships between researchers and participants (Goering et al., 2008). There are also several personal reasons why you might choose to disseminate this way and Johnson (2008) suggests three:

1. Writing stimulates clear thinking, discipline and a sense of accomplishment.
2. Writing can help develop your career and is a major determinant of promotion.
3. Writing can help develop the reputation of your institution.

To produce an article there are several decisions needed before starting to write. Cunningham (2004) recommends that you ask yourself two questions:

1. Is this research sufficient to generate interest by the profession?
2. What is an appropriate place to publish? (Consider also the impact factor[1] of the journal).

We suggest you look at Table 15.1 for practical tips when planning, Table 15.2 for writing and Table 15.3 for specific issues.

Table 15.1 Practical tips for planning (Creswell, 2005)

Tip	Description
Familiarise yourself with your chosen journal.	Understanding the aims and scope of the journal will help you see what types of articles are preferred.
Read journal articles.	Looking at published papers in the journal helps you assess how your work can follow a similar format.
Follow the journal guidelines.	When writing the article it is essential to take into account all editorial instructions. Look on the journal website and follow the 'instructions for authors' section; these are highly prescriptive and there is no room for negotiation.
Check costs.	It is important to check if there is a fee to publish in that journal.

---

[1]The impact factor of a journal is a measure which indicates the average number of citations to recent articles published. It is used as a way of indicating the importance of the journal relative to other journals.

Table 15.2   Practical tips for writing

Tip	Description
Start writing.	It may sound obvious, but start writing your paper as soon as you have your idea (Bourne, 2005).
Take one step at a time.	When preparing to publish take small incremental steps to prevent feelings of being overwhelmed (Cleary & Walter, 2004).
Originality of work.	The manuscript should be original and any copyright-protected material needs permission granted (Holmes et al., 2009).
Submit a single article to one journal only.	You must never send your paper to more than one journal at a time. Only if your manuscript is rejected can you revise it and send it elsewhere (Akyol, 2008).

Table 15.3   Specific writing issues for a paper

Tip	Description
Avoid jargon.	Avoid using jargon and write in a clear and accessible way (Cunningham, 2004).
Spelling and grammar.	There is no excuse for poor grammar and spelling errors as there are spell check functions on most computers (Cunningham, 2004).
Numbers in text.	Numbers one to nine should be spelled out in full, but numbers 10 and over can be in digit form. A sentence should never be started with a number in digit form (Cunningham, 2004).
First versus third person voice.	Many writers write in a detached third-person voice but this is contrary to the qualitative approach. Writing in the third-person style mutes the voices of the participants and of the author (Gilgun, 2005).
Remember the word limit.	All journals have word limits and medical journals particularly tend to have short word limits which are more challenging for qualitative research (Rowan, 1997).

Before you submit your article put yourself in the position of the reviewer and critically read through your paper. Remember that reviewers will be assessing the quality of the paper, the overall structure and presentation, the rigour of the methods and the appropriateness of the design. Reviewers will ask questions about the quality of the analysis, wanting to know what was done, by whom and how (Kuper et al., 2008). When you have redrafted enough times and are happy with the paper then it is useful to have one of your colleagues read through it.

 Do not be surprised if you get lots of feedback and try not to be offended.

A   **Activity   Critique your draft**

Go back to Chapter 4 and apply the steps of critiquing a journal article to your own draft. See what kind of comments you would make.

Dealing with the review process

When you have submitted your paper, the editor will decide whether to send it out to reviewers, although some may reject at this stage. Reviewers ask lots of questions during the process and Creswell (2005) highlights the most common:

- Whether the abstract is informative and concise.
- Whether the paper has the right appeal for the journal.
- Whether the research contributes new innovative insight.
- Whether there is sufficient context and focus in the argument.
- Whether the objectives are clearly laid out.
- Whether there is scientific rigour in the methodology.
- Whether the findings are well presented and transparent.
- Whether the references are accurate.
- Whether the paper is well written and well presented.
- What the main strengths and weaknesses are.

You may have to deal with rejection if the editors decide not to publish your article. There are many possible reasons for this. You may have failed to address an important issue, the paper may lack originality, the methodology may be inappropriate, or it may not be well written (Greenhalgh, 1997). Whilst you may feel that not all the comments are justified it is useful to take some time away and come back to your paper when you feel more emotionally able to deal with it. Try not to give up as you can now submit the paper to a different journal and use the comments to make your paper better.

Personal case example: Rejection and acceptance

We are not strangers to rejection ourselves. No matter how experienced you become you will still face criticism. We have received many reviews, ranging from positive or constructively critical to unhelpful, with some reviewers simply not understanding the specialised methods we used or having little tolerance for qualitative approaches. We have also had fair rejections where, with hindsight, we were able to reflect and see why the paper was not good enough for publication at that time, in that journal. Below we provide you with some examples. We do not directly quote the reviewers but instead give an impression of the type of things said.

Example

This paper discusses an important topic and has some potential to make a useful contribution to the field. It is does however have a number of shortcomings that need to be addressed. The reviewer went on to list several issues and lists eight references they felt were missing from the paper. This therefore required a substantial rewrite, but with the reviewer's help was a much better paper when it was published.

Example

This paper is easy to read and very interesting [...] the only query I have is ... This review was quite short as the reviewer felt that the paper was well written and needed very little revision.

Example

I feel that this paper would be better submitted to a journal that is focused on teaching as it does not fit with the scope of this journal. This paper was rejected by the journal and quite substantive feedback was given in relation to how to make improvements. It was disheartening but with hindsight we probably did choose the wrong journal.

How to prepare a conference presentation/poster

In the field of health there is a growing expectation that professionals should present their research at conferences (Cleary & Walter, 2004). Presenting a paper at a conference is an important way to disseminate knowledge to clinical audiences (Coad & Devitt, 2006), as well as to other professionals such as teachers or social workers. Presenting can be rewarding and conferences also provide opportunities for researchers and practitioners to exchange views (Lowcay & McIntyre, 2005).

The abstract

To be given the opportunity to present at a conference you will be expected to submit an abstract. Writing an abstract for a conference has three main purposes as outlined by Gordner and Burkett (2012):

1. To allow the conference committee to determine whether the research is relevant or not and make judgements about the writing quality.
2. Information in the abstract helps conference organisers arrange presentations and posters into themes.
3. Printed abstracts are distributed to delegates allowing them to decide which presentations to attend and which posters to view.

When you start your abstract you should begin by consulting the guidelines on the conference website. These will provide you with information about expectations and word limits (Gordner & Burkett, 2012). It is important to recognise that all abstracts are not the same but there is a general template for clinical paper abstracts which is outlined by Happell (2009):

- In the first couple of sentences give a short and clear description of the importance of the topic.
- Follow this with the setting and the participant demographics.
- Develop the process of how the programme or initiative was implemented with reference to any specific issues encountered.
- State the main results/findings.
- Draw the abstract to a close with some consideration of implications for mental health practice. It is important not to use blanket statements here but actually show what the findings mean and how they might be translated.
- In the conclusion of the abstract, provide an overview of the focus of the proposed presentation.

 Usually many more abstracts are submitted than are accepted and your abstract needs to represent more than just a good idea (Happell, 2007).

Preparing your oral presentation

If your abstract is accepted for an oral presentation then you need to prepare an interesting talk! Oral presentations help build your professional profile and disseminate your work. A key to good presentation lies with the slides that you prepare, which are often in PowerPoint format. Ranse and Hayes (2009) provide a useful overview, shown in Table 15.4.

Table 15.4   Preparing slides (Ranse & Hayes, 2009)

Slide	Description
Title	Include the names of the authors and convey the main message.
Overview	Indicate the progression of the presentation and be brief.
Background	Outline the current literature and provide a rationale for the research.
Aims	Indicate what you hope to achieve. We recommend that you are clear how your research might help children and families.
Findings	Present the methods and findings of the study.
Conclusion	Summarise the key points and orient the recommendations to the applied nature of the research.

This template serves as a guide to the nature of the slides for your presentation but is not prescriptive. You may wish to insert extra slides with additional information but be careful not to have too many. Remember, the audience has come to hear you talk about your research, not read it from a screen. Consider the following advice:

1. Have a sensible number of slides. Five is about right for a ten-minute presentation (Ranse & Hayes, 2009).
2. Ensure your font size is large enough to be visible from the back of the room, approximately size 24 (Happell, 2009).
3. Avoid your slides becoming too busy or overly detailed.
4. Acknowledge the people who have helped you (Ranse & Hayes, 2009).
5. Make your presentation visually appealing and if appropriate insert photos, movie clips, graphics or colour. Do not overuse images or colour as these do not necessarily impart knowledge and the goal of the presentation is to inform (Cleary & Walter, 2004).
6. Check with the conference organisers that your slide presentation is compatible with their software (Ranse & Hayes, 2009), particularly if you have used video or photos.
7. Take a copy of your presentation slides with you on the day, even if you have emailed in advance (Ranse & Hayes, 2009). It is also useful to take a printout of your slides to familiarise yourself with their order.
8. For smaller audiences it can be useful to have a hand-out available.
9. Make sure that your contact details are on the first or last slide so that people can contact you after the presentation if they want more details. It is also useful to include your project web address if you have one.

To help you think about how you present to an audience we provide practical advice in Table 15.5.

Table 15.5 Some dos and don'ts of presenting

Do	Don't
Introduce yourself to the chairperson on the day of your presentation so they know who you are (Ranse & Hayes, 2009).	Arrive late and forget to let the chairperson know that you are one of the presenters.
Be careful to maintain eye contact with your audience (Happell, 2009).	Simply read from your notes in a monotone voice and forget your audience is there!
Make sure you keep to time in your presentation (Happell, 2009). The chairperson will help you with this.	Ignore the chairperson's gestures or signs that you are running out of time
Learn from others. It is a good idea to attend one or two presentations as a delegate before you present one.	Compare yourself to others. Experienced presenters who are confident and familiar with the materials may come across very well and this may make you have unrealistic expectations regarding what you can do.
Have a glass of water available in case you get a dry throat from anxiety (Happell, 2009).	Let anxiety block you from attending and presenting at conferences. Use whatever anxiety reduction techniques you can to alleviate it.

Preparing your poster

Posters are an effective way to disseminate and can be a good place to start if you have not presented at a conference before. Demands for oral presentations are high and you may have more opportunity to submit a poster when there are limited oral slots. As with all forms of dissemination there will be clear guidelines provided by the conference organisers regarding the most appropriate way to produce your poster, so make sure you follow them. These guidelines will tell you whether to present your poster in landscape or portrait orientation, how many words you can use and what size your overall poster should be (Lowcay and McIntyre, 2005).

There are several principles that apply to designing any poster:

1. Look at other people's posters before you start, to get an idea of what you think looks good and what you would avoid doing.
2. Sketch out roughly how you would like to design your poster and where you would place text boxes or illustrations.
3. When you start to translate your design onto a computer, bear in mind that you are likely to be designing it on A4 size. However, the finished poster will be considerably larger, so remember this when deciding your font size. Also, for any pictures, photographs or graphics that you include, ensure that they are of a high enough pixel density to still look crisp and clear when enlarged.
4. Remember your layout and formatting needs to be accurate; for example if you have text boxes, make sure that they line up perfectly, as tiny

variations will look much worse when the poster is enlarged. It is usually best to stick to about three different sizes of font and it is likely to look smarter and more professional if you stick to two colours.

5. Use a mixture of text and pictures and be really selective about what you include.

6. A poster is a very concise representation of your research and it is impossible to include all of the information that you may think is important. You can always have paper copies with more information about your research to give to interested viewers.

Once you have designed your poster, ask colleagues to proof read it. Any mistakes will be magnified when the poster is enlarged. Check that you have your name, the names of any affiliates or sponsors on the poster with the correct logos and your email address for correspondence. When you have double-checked everything, you are ready to send your design to the printer to be enlarged and laminated; there will be a fee for this, so get your poster right before it is printed! Remember to factor in the time it will take for your poster to be created, so that you have plenty of time to collect it.

 Any tiny mistakes in designing your poster will be magnified when printed at a larger size.

Workshops

Workshops are often organised to help develop the skills of delegates and provide some training centred round a particular issue or subject. These may be data sessions, during which participants discuss a particular data set and contribute towards the analysis. Alternatively it may be an arena to communicate recommendations generated from a particular piece of research. You may be invited or volunteer to run a workshop based on your research to inform others of the findings and recommendations for practice. Your audiences may comprise:

- People from your participant group.
- People from your organisation.
- Clinical/education/social care professionals.
- Managers, commissioners, funding bodies.
- Academic audiences (typically conferences have workshop slots attached to their schedules).
- Other groups to whom your findings may be relevant (e.g. voluntary sector workers).

Workshops have an instructor (which will be you) and a small number of delegates. Typically workshops last from half-day to full-day and require active participation. Workshops tend to emphasise a discussion round a theme and involve the delegates engaging in activities.

How to run a workshop

When you are planning your workshop you need to remain mindful that it will require you to be organised and focused, leaving scope for a lot of creative thinking. You need clear objectives about what you are aiming to achieve from the workshop before you start. Workshops are useful for building relationships, networking, problem solving and for offering new ideas and training.

 Remember that you are not delivering a lecture but facilitating a discussion.

When you plan your workshop there are a number of areas you need to plan in advance:

- Define your goals and be clear on your objectives.
- Decide on the key audiences and invite the appropriate people to attend.
- Set an agenda and give all participants a copy.
- Have a copy of any reports written on the research for delegates to take away.

When running your workshop there are a number of things you need to be mindful of:

- Break the ice at the start so that people have time to get to know one another.
- Be aware that some people may be nervous interacting with others they do not know so when planning group exercises keep the group small.
- Make sure you have appropriate materials available for each of your groups (pens, paper).
- Allow time at the end of each activity to share ideas.
- Enjoy the process.
- Ensure all delegates have your contact details.

How to write a thesis/dissertation

If you are undertaking your research project for an educational qualification then you are likely to be required to submit a thesis/dissertation. The nature of your qualification and level of study will determine the word length. Some undergraduate level courses set a word limit of approximately 6000 words, Master's level may vary from 12000–20000 words, whereas Doctorate level may be as high as 80000 words.

Writing a thesis/dissertation is similar to writing a paper. Nonetheless your thesis/dissertation will probably be longer than an article and will require more detail. You need to ensure that you consult the guidelines produced by your educational establishment and communicate regularly with your supervisor. As a general rule the thesis/dissertation is broken down under a number of headings. The first part is outlined in Table 15.6, the main body is outlined in Table 15.7 and final sections are in Table 15.8.

Table 15.6   First sections

Section	Description
The title page	This should include all of your details, and the research title should be original, interesting and capture your reader's attention.
Acknowledgements	It is likely that you will need the support of several people as you progress through your research and you will rely on the involvement of your participants. It is important to thank all of these people (without compromising the anonymity of your participants).
Contents page	A clear table of contents and a contents list of figures and tables is needed.
Abstract	Typically this shows what you did, what you found and what you concluded, including the implications of those findings.

Table 15.7   Main body

Section	Description
Introduction/ background/literature review	This section provides the context for your research and highlights the limits and gaps in current evidence. This provides a platform for presenting an argument for how your research adds to existing knowledge. It can be helpful to break up this argument using signposts and illustrate clearly the implications and impact for children with mental health difficulties.
Methods	This is an important chapter in your thesis/dissertation. All of your methodological choices should be outlined with a rationale. Remember that you will need to demonstrate clearly how you have managed ethical concerns.
Results/findings	In this chapter you report your findings or results. For qualitative research it is likely that you will have more than one findings chapter and you will need to provide detailed analysis.
Discussion	In this chapter you need to contextualise your findings within the broader context and literature whilst also summarising your key findings. It will be necessary to make clear links with the existing evidence. For a qualitative project you will also need a strong section on reflexivity here.

Table 15.8   Final sections

Section	Description
References	Your references list should conform to the guidelines and should be fairly substantial.
Appendices	You are likely to submit an appendices section with a blank copy of your consent form, information sheet, proposal, pilot study summary, letters of invitation and any other useful information.

Starting writing

Writing requires practice and skills which are often only given limited attention in clinical training (Parry, 1996). Getting started can be difficult and writer's block is a common experience. It can be helpful to take a few minutes to think about what is blocking you and if necessary take a short break (Murray, 2006). Remember you are not aiming for perfection and in the early stages you just need to write. Drafting and redrafting is essential. Try not to write the whole chapter as this can be difficult. Instead aim to write one of the sub-sections based on your notes and reading.

Whenever you refer to the work of others, whether in your own words or directly quoted it is essential that you reference it appropriately. If you are found to have plagiarised the work of someone else in your thesis/dissertation then there are likely to be serious consequences including being dismissed from the course and/or discredited (Murray, 2006).

 Remember that plagiarism is <u>NOT</u> acceptable and your examiners are likely to notice if you have plagiarised the work of others.

Using the internet for dissemination

The internet allows many different audiences, including the general public, access to reports, articles and presentations, which is particularly important if the research was publicly funded (Duffy, 2000). However, disseminating qualitative findings online requires some expertise (Keen and Todres, 2007). There are different ways of doing this and often your work will be posted on websites by others. For example, many journals are now 'open access' which allows papers to be viewed by a broad audience. Often conference organisers will post abstracts on their websites and it is sometimes possible for a copy of your presentation to be included. Alternatively you can write your own research blog to attach to your own website or your organisation's web page so that others can view your work.

Disseminating through the internet can be appealing as it is cost-effective and reaches a wider audience. However, you do need to think about which audience you wish to reach as not everyone has access to the internet, particularly in certain countries. Nonetheless it is a quick, flexible method which can raise the profile of your organisation and supplement other methods of writing.

Leaflets

Information leaflets are sometimes desirable to disseminate practical messages from your research. Ultimately the format/content of these leaflets will depend on who you are producing them for. In child mental health you may either want to produce information leaflets based on your findings for children themselves, or for families or professionals.

The skill of producing a good leaflet is to convey the message clearly and succinctly. The leaflet should be attractive so that readers are encouraged to read the contents and (if funds permit) colour is helpful. The language should be simple, avoiding jargon. Remember that if you use abbreviations you need to spell out their meaning as your audience may not be familiar with them (O'Reilly et al., 2013). It can be helpful with leaflets for a particular group to enlist service users for advice about the final wording or format of your leaflet to ensure that the language is accessible and clear.

Reports

Many organisations have an annual report for organisational use, promoting the organisation or public release. You may be able to include your research within this report to showcase your work and report your key findings. This is a useful way of contributing to your organisation and helping raise its profile. Depending on how much space you have available it is necessary to report the key literature, the main methodological choices, the core findings and a critical discussion to contextualise them. Do not forget to thank your participants and any gatekeepers, while maintaining their anonymity.

Alternatively you may need to produce a report of your own to report your research for your organisation or other audiences. This is often a requirement for funding bodies so they may have a particular structure or style that you are expected to follow. Nonetheless, make sure you keep the layout simple and use a language which is appropriate and accessible to the reader. Keep the main messages of the report simple and where appropriate use images or graphics to make the report more appealing. It is always a good idea to look at reports written by others so that you can judge what does or does not work well. It is also a good idea to have an electronic copy on your organisation's website.

This is a useful forum to express the recommendations you have made from your findings.

Press releases and media

Press releases can be a good way of raising awareness. This can be important if the area of child mental health you are researching has a high impact on children and families.

 In some organisations it is mandatory to consult with the media/ communications office in the preparation of a press release (O'Reilly et al., 2013).

For illustration purposes we provide an example press release. A student at the University of Leicester, Elizabeth Hale, was interested in children's experiences of caring for a parent with inflammatory arthritis with an objective of developing educational resources for them.

The press release can be accessed through the following web link: www. arthritisresearchuk.org/news/press-releases/2012/december/researchers-to-develop-educational-resources-to-help-families-affected-by-arthritis.aspx

We have provided a copy of the press release here (Figure 15.1) to give an idea of the visual layout, but you may want to visit the website. We thank Arthritis Research UK (www.arthritisresearchuk.org) for allowing us to reproduce this.

Other effective ways of using the media for dissemination are through newspapers, magazines, television and radio. This can be anxiety provoking and there is the risk that you may lose some control over what is said about your research. To promote your findings through these media outlets, it is worth getting training in this area and advice from others. Nonetheless good local or national coverage can promote your personal profile and get your research message out to those who need it most.

 When disseminating through the media make sure that your participants cannot be identified.

Although you may not actively decide to use the media to disseminate your work, publishing through other means does open your research up to being

Researcher to develop educational resources to help families affected by arthritis

Published on 21 December 2012

Researchers in Dudley, funded by Arthritis Research UK, are aiming to produce information about arthritis aimed at children whose parents are living with the painful condition.

Elizabeth Hale, based at Russells Hall Hospital, has been awarded £30,000 from medical research charity Arthritis Research UK to find out what kind of information could be useful to youngsters aged between seven and eleven years, whose mother or father is affected by inflammatory arthritis.

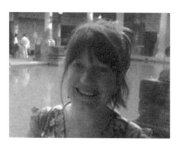

Ms Hale, a health psychologist for The Dudley Group NHS Foundation Trust, will collaborate with colleagues at the University of Leicester to build on earlier research which suggests that adults with inflammatory arthritis find it difficult to speak to their children about their condition.

One in six people in the UK are affected by arthritis but many parents worry that discussing this with their children could be upsetting to them.

Through interviewing a number of families over two years, the study will examine how parents and children talk to one another about arthritis, focusing particularly on the child's perceptions of the condition.

It is hoped that the study will highlight the need for development of educational resources targeted specifically at children aged seven to eleven years, while providing insight about how, when and by whom this information should be delivered.

Ms Hale said: "Being diagnosed with inflammatory arthritis such as rheumatoid arthritis, ankylosing spondylitis, psoriatic arthritis or lupus, is an unsettling prospect for any patient, but the impact it can also have on their children should not be underestimated. Children are likely to be anxious about their parents' welfare and this worry could easily have a negative impact on their lives, affecting schoolwork or causing behavioural changes.

"Developing a range of appropriate educational resources could play a vital role in helping children to better understand their parents' condition and empower them to ask questions that they might otherwise be nervous about asking. Equally, providing parents with some guidelines about how to broach such a difficult subject could also be beneficial to the overall psychological well-being of the family."

Ms Hale currently works both on a one-to-one basis and in group settings with patients who have a range of rheumatic diseases. She has developed an education programme for patients with early rheumatoid arthritis, which has input from the multidisciplinary rheumatology team.

Professor Panos Vostanis, of the University of Leicester's School of Psychology, said: "The needs of children of parents with a chronic physical illness are often not recognised, consequently are not being met by appropriate services. Such recognition and understanding requires evidence based on children's perceptions and experiences.

"Michelle O'Reilly and I are building on previous studies with children of different ages in the collaborative study with Elizabeth Hale from Dudley NHS Trust, towards her PsyD at the University of Leicester."

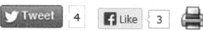

Figure 15.1   Press release

accessed by the media. Sometimes correspondents from news media attend academic/clinical conferences or may learn about your research from funding bodies, websites or journal articles. It is possible that you may be contacted by someone to present your expertise on a particular area of child mental health. Do not accept immediately but give yourself some time to think about it. If you decide to go ahead, it is important that you work as closely as you can with them so as to not be misrepresented. Make sure you plan carefully what you are going to say in advance.

Ethics of dissemination

Disseminating your research is not a straightforward process and it is important to remember that there are some ethical considerations in writing-up. These include:

- Not wasting the time of your participants by failing to use the data.
- Protecting their identity.
- Making sure that the findings are accessible.
- Reporting negative findings.
- Declaring conflicts of interest.
- Ensuring that your work is transparent.

Not wasting time: It is important not to waste your participants' time. There is little point spending time with each child if you have little intention of sharing your findings beyond your own needs. During the planning stages of your research you should have outlined your objectives, including dissemination proposals.

Protecting identity: When you start publishing your work there is a risk that others who know the participants will recognise the anecdotes, stories, experiences or 'voices' of those children. Although you do not want to lose the richness of the data or the quality of the interpretations you do need to exercise care in how much is revealed through a specific quotation. A good example of this was data collected in a small village. When it was disseminated some members of the community were able to deduce who was being referred to, which created some distress (Stein, 2010).

 A   **Activity   Deductive disclosure**

We recommend you read this paper as it details some of the issues with representation and deductive disclosure and provides a personal account of the problems encountered.

(Continued)

(Continued)

Stein, A. (2010). Sex, truths, and audiotape: Anonymity and the ethics of public exposure in ethnography. *Journal of Contemporary Ethnography*, *39*(5), 554–568.

Making findings accessible: You have an ethical responsibility to ensure your findings are accessible to the intended audience. There is little point writing in academic language if you are writing for children and similarly it may be unhelpful to use academic terminology if you are writing for practitioners. Policy makers and commissioners will need to appreciate the core messages being transmitted and a translation of findings will be essential. Also, the general public may be interested in your findings but will need this in a format they can understand (Oliver, 2010).

Reporting negative findings: You may be disappointed initially not to find what you thought you might. Nonetheless it is important you write this up. If you do not, money and time may be wasted again on more research looking at the effects of that intervention, not knowing that the results have already been found. In qualitative research you might find that children and families have very negative views of services of treatments or of professionals but it is still important that these voices are given a chance to be heard.

Declare conflicts of interest: Often during the dissemination process, particularly in journals, you will be asked this anyway but it is important to be mindful of what they are. The most obvious conflict of interest is the funding source but there are others. For example if you work for a particular mental health service and your participants say negative things it may have implications for you in how you disseminate that information. You need to be careful to be transparent about any conflicts you have.

Transparency: To be ethical you need to be transparent. When writing up your findings it is important that you are clear about what you did, what you found, on what basis you made your interpretations and what you concluded. It should be clear to the reader how you did your research and how you drew your conclusions.

Sharing findings with participants

A common complaint by participant communities is that research teams forget about them once the data are collected (Dixon-Woods et al., 2011). This is potentially because there are issues relating to how research findings might be shared with participants and how this links with the methodological goals and ethical standards in healthcare research (Goldblatt et al., 2011).

Giving feedback to children and parents

When disseminating to families be clear about the ethical boundaries of the feedback. You can give general feedback from the project as a whole and ensure that any references to data are anonymous, but be aware that deductive disclosure may occur if parents know each other or if something specific identifies a child to their parent. Remember that you have promised the children anonymity and unless they have shared the information with their parents they may not want you to. Evidence suggests that many parents feel they have the right to be offered the research findings (Fernandez et al., 2009) and so you may have to handle this delicately if the child prefers you not to do so.

 There are possibly some negative implications of sharing the findings/ results with research participants as some may find it emotionally distressing (Markham, 2006).

Deciding on the format of feedback

A fundamental issue when providing feedback to children is presenting it in a format that they understand. It is important that the children appreciate the key messages and are able to assimilate that information. You may decide that an oral presentation for the group of participants is a useful way to convey the message. Alternatively you may provide each child with a leaflet, email or poster.

For parents you may want to provide feedback separately. The information leaflet or poster designed for the children is not likely to be sufficient for their parents. You could send out separate emails to each parent or write a short letter outlining the main findings. Alternatively a more personal touch may be to make a telephone call to each parent so that they have the opportunity to ask you questions. Again if ethics permit it may be a good idea to present the overall findings face-to-face with a group of parents with a more interactive style to disseminate the overall messages.

Member-checking

Typically sharing research findings with participants for methodological and ethical reasons is referred to as member-check (Goldblatt et al., 2011). Member-check is a process whereby the researcher goes back to the participants to check whether the explanations and interpretations resonate with the participant, reflecting what they felt, said, meant or expressed (Merriam, 2002). By using member-check the researcher is able to provide feedback to participants but also get something back from them. By checking the interpretations there is the potential to reduce incorrect or distorted data transcription and interpretation (Goldblatt et al., 2011).

 Member-checking is not a suitable modality of authentication for some qualitative approaches, particularly those that are relativist. This would oppose the ontology.

Professional case example   Interview with Professor Dogra and Dr Svirydzenka

Professor Nisha Dogra and Dr Nadzeya Svirydzenka (University of Leicester) have conducted studies with children and provided feedback of the findings. We asked them some questions about the challenges of disseminating to children.

What do you think the challenges are of disseminating your findings to children?

The initial barrier would be convincing adults that children should have the information. Mental health is, at times, seen as a sensitive subject to discuss with children due to the lack of awareness on the benefits these discussions can have. Therefore, involving adults in having these discussions is the first challenge. When it comes to the methods of actually making research results available to children, one needs to consider how to make the findings relevant to children and also making them user friendly. If you do that, children will be more likely to engage with the material.

What do you think is best practice for giving feedback to children?

When giving the information to children it is important to use age appropriate language and use a range of dissemination methods. It is also important to be prepared to discuss your findings and their implications. Hopefully, you have discussed these issues with the children that took part in your research and therefore discussing your findings with them would fall on eager ears. Branching out to include the general population of children and young people and raising mental health awareness needs to come in child-friendly language and format, as well as with clearly defined outcomes that will directly affect or be relevant to them. Using these techniques will not only help disseminate your results, but also carry an educational aspect in promoting good mental health.

How did the children from your project respond to receiving your disseminated findings?

Dissemination of our findings was done in the schools where the study took place. Our findings were presented by teachers and support staff in a way that related to their curriculum in mental health and well-being, which therefore made the format of dissemination relevant to an educational side of the findings. Young people valued seeing how the findings related to them and their school, since they themselves or their classmates have taken part in the study.

Some useful references

Vostanis, P., Svirydzenka, N., Dugard, P., Singh, S.P. & Dogra, N. (in press). Mental health service use by adolescents of Indian and White origin. *Archives of Disease in Childhood.*

Dogra, N., Svirydzenka, N., Dugard, P., Singh, S.P. & Vostanis, P. (in press). The characteristics and rates of mental health problems among Indian and White adolescents in two English cities. *British Journal of Psychiatry.*

Translating and implementing research into practice

Although we have demonstrated the importance of dissemination for practice, it might be easy to think that the relationship between evidence and practice is straightforward. However, there are several challenges to translating knowledge into practice. Implementing the changes indicated by research into clinical/educational contexts requires professionals to examine the process of transferring knowledge and skills within their local context.

There is still little literature published that addresses what is known as the 'translational research agenda' (Brekke et al., 2007). In other words, there is little guidance for practitioners or researchers regarding how to bridge the gap between published research and real-world practice. To translate evidence into a specific aspect of care requires more than simply identifying quality evidence. What is also needed is an assessment of relevance, organisational fit and resources (Rycroft-Malone et al., 2004). An additional difficulty relates to the limited uptake of conclusions from qualitative studies by policy makers and commissioners in their decision-making dialogue (Thorne, 2009). In health, there are differing perspectives regarding the principles and practicalities of adopting an evidence-based approach. These have been considered by a range of different authors from different disciplines, as outlined below:

1. Professionals struggle to keep pace with the rapid advances in health-care knowledge (Grol & Grimshaw, 2003).
2. There may be a lack of accessibility to findings (Small, 2005).
3. There are many important questions about mental health that remain unanswered (Waddell & Godderis, 2005).
4. The clinical environment is often not conducive to change (Grol & Grimshaw, 2003).
5. The evidence-based movement favours quantitative evidence yielded from randomised controlled trials but real professionals require evidence to address efficacy in typical practice settings (Waddell & Godderis, 2005).
6. A lack of cultural understanding may mean that the findings are not understood by those with limited training in research methods (Small, 2005).
7. Research is often cited as a way of limiting services and dictating the way they are funded and managed by organisations which suggests that evidence is being used too narrowly by policy makers (Waddell & Godderis, 2005).
8. Clinical professionals are often sceptical about evidence-based practice (Wadell & Godderis, 2005).

It is arguable that children's mental health services typically fail to reflect best-practice as suggested by the evidence available, which means that it is essential that the evidence-based agenda is engaged with by practitioners if children's mental health is to be improved (Hoagwood et al., 2001). Remember that evidence-based practice for child mental health is different from adult mental health. Because children undergo rapid physiological, neurological and psychological changes over a briefer period than adults, evidence-based practice needs to account for these developmental conditions, which may affect research and services (Hoagwood et al., 2001).

 A   Activity   Challenges of implementation

To help you to reflect on your own ideas about evidence-based practice we suggest that you write your own list of the challenges you may face in disseminating your findings so that they are useful to practitioners.

You may have noticed some changes in the field of child mental health with regards to how researchers engage in partnerships with policy makers and practitioners in designing their projects. In addition more practitioners are now able to carry out their own research projects with new initiatives for encouraging research within healthcare.

Summary

This chapter has introduced you to the most popular forms of research dissemination. Throughout the chapter we have provided you with practical tips on how to produce a journal article, conference presentations and posters. This has included practical guidance for preparing the abstract and the presentation slides. This chapter has introduced you to some of the alternative forms of dissemination, including writing a thesis/dissertation, internet, leaflets and the media, with consideration of their benefits and limitations within child mental health. We provided you with guidance on how to use these different dissemination practices before leading onto discussing the ethics of writing-up, including considerations in sharing your research findings with your participants and their parents. The chapter concluded with a presentation of the challenges of implementing research in practice.

Key messages

- Journal articles are a credible, peer-reviewed way of disseminating your research.
- Presenting at conferences can help you reach interested audiences.
- A thesis or dissertation is typically longer than a journal article and is written for academic qualification assessments.
- Sharing your research findings with participants is desirable but needs to be handled carefully.

Further reading

Cresswell, J. (2005). *Writing for academic success: A postgraduate guide*. London: Sage.

Johnson, T. (2008). Tips on how to write a paper. *Journal American Academy Dermatology*, *59*(6), 1064–1069.

Murray, R. (2006). *How to write a thesis* (Second edition). Berkshire: Open University Press.

GLOSSARY

Altruism   refers to putting the needs of another before one's own; selflessness.

Asymmetry   refers to two parts not being the same or equal. This links with a power imbalance.

Audit   a process whereby the auditor measures current practice against a set of standards which have been predefined. Its aim is to establish the extent to which actual practice compares with best practice.

Autonomy   refers to the individual having independence to make their own choices.

Beneficence   refers to the act or quality of being kind or doing good.

Capacity   refers to an individual's ability to make decisions, usually in relation to their developmental and intellectual abilities.

Coercion   the act of persuading an individual, or forcing them through unethical means.

Deductive disclosure   this refers to the risk in qualitative research of friends or colleagues of the participants in the data recognising those participants despite the quotations being anonymous.

Demographics   refers to the statistical data regarding the characteristics of your sample, such as their age, gender and race.

Dissemination   to disseminate your work means to distribute it so that others may read it.

Encryption   refers to the process of coding information so that it cannot be viewed by unauthorised persons. Typically this is achieved through passwords.

Epistemology   epistemology refers to the theory of knowledge and is concerned with what we know, how we know it and who knows it.

Exclusion criteria   the specific criteria the researcher decides to use to determine whether particular participants should be excluded from the study.

Exploitation   refers to the act of treating people unfairly or taking advantage of them.

Gatekeepers   the individuals who have some authority over the children the researcher may want to access. They have the power to grant or refuse access.

Generalisability   relates to the extent to which the findings are relevant and applicable to other members of the population.

Ideology   a set of ideas or beliefs that are considered important by a particular group or culture.

Inclusion criteria   the criteria that are specified by the research which must be present in the participant sample. These are the criteria by which the researcher decides whether a participant is eligible to be included in the study.

Likert scale   this is a form of asking questions on a questionnaire so that respondents rate their answers in terms of the strength of their agreement. This is a psychometric scale where respondents specify their level of agreement with a statement to capture the intensity of feelings.

Mental health   a state of being mentally healthy. Mental health refers to a general state of well-being and a freedom from mental illness.

Mental illness   an impairment of the person's capacity to function; the presence of a mental disorder or condition.

Mixed methods   a mixed methods design is one whereby the researcher uses both quantitative and qualitative methods in their approach. The results/findings from these two aspects are then combined, integrated or triangulated.

Naturally occurring   refers to collecting data from natural contexts whereby the event would continue to occur regardless of the involvement of the researcher.

Non-maleficence   the ethical principle referring to doing no harm to research participants.

Ontology   an underpinning philosophy, referring to the nature of reality.

Paradigm   a complicated term which is understood to have various meanings, but can be characterised as a set of beliefs which represent a particular world view.

Positivism   a position which assumes a relationship between the world and the understanding the research holds of it. It relates to the natural sciences, assuming that there is an objective reality which can be measured.

Qualitative research   qualitative research is used to explore people's beliefs, experiences and perceptions and is usually conducted with smaller sample sizes. It is concerned with depth of information.

Quantitative research   quantitative research is based upon scientific principles with an aim to generate large-scale numerical data so that the researcher may predict trends. Quantitative research starts with a hypothesis and seeks to generalise results to wider populations.

Rapport   the building of a positive relationship between two or more people.

Reflexivity   refers to the process of actively reflecting upon the role and impact that the researcher has had on the research process. This means that the researcher has to consider the influences upon the data collection and data analysis.

Reliability   refers to the extent to which the research study could be easily replicated by another researcher.

Social constructionism   a position that believes things do not pre-exist but that they are co-created in a social, historical and political context.

Therapeutic misconception   relates to when the participant is not able to understand the difference between the goals of the research and the goals of their treatment and may misunderstand that research does not necessarily have therapeutic benefit. This is particularly concerning in medical trials.

Transferability   the extent to which the findings from one qualitative research study can be transferred to other settings.

Validity   refers to the extent to which the researcher has managed to measure what they intended to measure in the study.

REFERENCES

Abiddin, N., Hassan, A. & Ahmad, A. (2009). Research student supervision: An approach to good supervisory practice. *The Open Education Journal, 2*, 11–16.

Ahmedani, B., Harold, R., Fitton, V. & Shifflet-Gibson, E. (2011). What adolescents can tell us: Technology and the future of social work education. *Social Work Education, 30*(7), 830–846.

Akyol, A. (2008). How to write a paper for publication. *International Journal of Human Sciences, 5*(2), online.

Alderson, P. (2004). Ethics. In S. Fraser, V. Lewis, S. Ding, M. Kellett & C. Robinson (eds), *Doing research with children and young people*. London: Sage.

Alderson, P. (2005). Designing ethical research with children. In A. Farrell (ed.), *Doing research with children and young people* (pp. 97–112). Thousand Oaks, CA: Sage.

Alderson, P. (2007). Governance and ethics in health research. In M. Saks & J. Allsop (eds), *Researching health: Qualitative, quantitative and mixed methods* (pp. 283–300). London: Sage.

Alderson, P. & Morrow, V. (2004). *Ethics, social research and consulting with children and young people*. Ilford: Barnardos.

Aldridge, J. (2007). Picture this: The use of participatory photographic research methods with people with learning disabilities. *Disability and Society, 22*(1), 1–17.

Antaki, C. & O'Reilly, M. (in press). Either/or questions in psychiatric assessments: The effect of the seriousness and order of the alternatives, *Discourse Studies*.

Atkinson, P. & Coffey, A. (2004). Analysing documentary realities. In D. Silverman (ed.), *Qualitative research: Theory, method and practice* (Second edition) (pp. 56–75). London: Sage.

Ayling, R. & Mewse, A. (2009). Evaluating internet interviews with gay men. *Qualitative Health Research, 19*, 566–576.

Baez, B. (2002). Confidentiality in qualitative research: Reflections on secrets, power and agency. *Qualitative Research, 2*(1), 35–58.

Bagley, S., Reynolds, W. & Nelson, R. (2007). Is a 'wage-payment' model for research participation appropriate for children? *Pediatrics, 119*(1), 46–51.

Barke, R. (2009). Balancing uncertain risks and benefits in human subjects research. *Science, Technology, and Human Values, 34*(3), 337–364.

Barter, C. & Renold, E. (2000). 'I wanna tell you a story': Exploring the application of vignettes in qualitative research with children and young people. *International Journal of Social Research Methodology, 3*(4), 307–323.

Beauchamp, T. & Childress, J. (2008). *Principles of Biomedical Ethics* (Sixth edition). Oxford: Oxford University Press.

Bell, A. (2007). Designing and testing questionnaires for children. *Journal of Research in Nursing, 12*(5), 461–469.

Bell, L. (1998). Public and private meanings in diaries, in researching family and childcare. In J. Ribbens & R. Edwards (eds), *Feminist dilemmas in qualitative research: Public knowledge and private lives* (pp. 72–86). London: Sage.

Benjamin, H. & MacKinlay, D. (2010). Communicating challenges: Overcoming disability. In S. Redsell & A. Hastings (eds), *Listening to children and young people in healthcare consultations* (pp. 151–168). Oxon: Radcliffe Publishing.

Beresford, B. (1997). *Personal accounts: Involving disabled children in research.* New York: Social Policy Research Unit.

Berger, R. & Paul, M. (2011). Using e-mail for family research. *Journal of Technology in Human Sciences, 29*, 197–211.

Bertrand, C. & Bordeau, L. (2010). Research interviews by Skype: A new data collection method. In J. Esteves (ed.), *Proceedings of the 9th European Conference on Research Methodology for Business and Management Studies* (pp. 70–79). Madrid: IE Business School.

Billig, M., Condor, S., Edwards, D., Gane, M., Middleton, D. & Radley, A. (1988). *Ideological dilemmas: A social psychology of everyday thinking.* London: Sage.

Black, N. (1992). The relationship between evaluative research and audit. *Journal of Public Health Medicine, 14*(4), 361–366.

Blaxter, L., Hughes, C. & Tight, M. (2001). *How to research* (Second edition). Buckingham: Open University Press.

Bloor, M., Fincham, B. & Sampson, H. (2007). Qualiti (NCRM) Commissioned inquiry into the risk to well-being of researchers in qualitative research. Cardiff: School of Social Sciences. www.cf.ac.uk/socsi/qualiti/CIReport.pdf.

Bloor, M., Fincham, B. & Sampson, H. (2010). Unprepared for the worst: Risks of harm for qualitative researchers. *Methodological Innovations, 5*(1), 45–55.

Bogolub, E. & Thomas, N. (2005). Parental consent and the ethics of research with foster children. *Qualitative Social Work, 4*(3), 271–292.

Bolger, N., Davis, A. & Rafaeli, E. (2003). Diary methods: Capturing life as it is lived. *Annual Review of Psychology, 54*, 579–616.

Borbasi, S., Chapman, Y. & Read, K. (2002). Perceptions of the researcher: In-depth interviewing in the home. *Contemporary Nurse, 14*(1), 24–37.

Bottorff, J. L. (1994). Using videotaped data recordings in qualitative research. In J. M. Morse (ed.), *Critical issues in qualitative research methods* (pp. 244–261). London: Sage.

Boud, D., Keogh, R. & Walker, D. (1985). *Reflection: Turning experience into learning*. London: Kogan Page.

Bourne, P. (2005). Ten simple rules for getting published. *PLoS Computational Biology, 1*(5), e57: 0341–0342.

Boyatzis, R. (1998). *Transforming qualitative information: Thematic analysis and code development*. London: Sage.

Brannen, J. (1998). Research note: The study of sensitive topics. *Sociological Review, 36*, 552–563.

Branthwaite, A. & Patterson, S. (2011). The power of qualitative research in the era of social media. *Qualitative Market Research: An International Journal, 14*(4), 430–440.

Braun, V. & Clarke, V. (2006). Using thematic analysis in psychology. *Qualitative Research in Psychology, 3*, 77–101.

Brekke, J., Ell, K. & Palinkas, L. (2007). Translational science at the National Institute of Mental Health: Can social work take its rightful place? *Research on Social Work Practice, 17*(1), 123–133.

Britten, N. (2000). Qualitative interviews in health care research. In C. Pope & N. Mays (eds), *Qualitative research in health care* (pp. 11–19). London: BMJ Books.

Bromley, J., Hare, D., Davison, K. & Emerson, E. (2004). Mothers supporting children with autistic spectrum disorders: social support, mental health status and satisfaction with services. *Autism, 8*(4), 409–423.

Bryman, A. (2008). *Social research methods* (Third edition). Oxford: Oxford University Press.

Burgess, R. (1981). Keeping a research diary. *Cambridge Journal of Education, 11*(1), 75–83.

Burns, E. (2010). Developing email interview practices in qualitative research. *Sociological Research Online, 15*(4), Art 8, *[online journal]*. Retrieved from www. socresonline.org.uk/15/4/8.html on 15 February 2013.

Burr, V. (1995). *An introduction to social constructionism*. London: Routledge.

Busch, S. & Barry, C. (2007). Mental health disorders in childhood: Assessing the burden on families. *Health Affairs, 26*(4), 1088–1095.

Bushin, N. (2007). Interviewing children in their homes: Putting ethical principles into practice and developing flexible techniques. *Children's Geographies, 5*(3), 235–251.

Butz, A. & Alexander, C. (1991). Use of health diaries with children. *Nursing Research, 40*(1), 59–61.

Cahill, P. & Papageorgiou, A. (2007). Video analysis of communication in paediatric consultations in primary care. *British Journal of General Practice, 57*, 866–871.

Cameron, H. (2005). Asking the tough questions: A guide to ethical practices in interviewing young children. *Early Child Development and Care, 175*(6), 597–610.

Carroll, K., Iedema, R. & Kerridge, R. (2008). Reshaping ICU ward round practices using video-reflexive ethnography. *Qualitative Health Research, 18*(3), 380–390.

Carter, B. (2009). Tick box for child? The ethical positioning of children as vulnerable, researchers as barbarians and reviewers as overly cautious. *International Journal of Nursing Studies, 46*, 858–864.

Charmaz, K. (2005). Grounded theory in the 21st century: Applications for advancing social justice studies. In N. Denzin & Y. Lincoln (eds), *The SAGE handbook of qualitative research* (Third edition) (pp. 507–535). London: Sage.

Charmaz, K. (2006). *Constructing grounded theory: Practical guide through qualitative analysis.* London: Sage.

Chenail, R. (2011). Qualitative researchers in the Blogosphere: Using blogs as diaries and data. *The Qualitative Report, 16*(1), 249–254.

Chorpita, B. & Regan, J. (2009). Dissemination of effective mental health treatment procedures: Maximizing the return on a significant investment. *Behaviour Research and Therapy, 47*(11), 990–993.

Christensen, P. (2004). Children's participation in ethnographic research: Issues of power and representation, *Children and Society, 18*, 165–176.

Clark, A. (2005). Listening to and involving young children: A review of research and practice. *Early Child Development and Care, 175*(6), 489–505.

Cleary, M. & Walter, G. (2004). Apportioning our time and energy: Oral presentation, poster, journal article or other? *International Journal of Mental Health Nursing, 13*, 204–207.

Closs, S. & Cheater, F. (1996). Audit or research – what is the difference? *Journal of Clinical Nursing, 5*, 249–256

Coad, J. & Devitt, P. (2006). Research dissemination: The art of writing an abstract for conferences. *Nurse Education in Practice, 6*(2), 112–116.

Coad, J. & Lewis, A. (2004). *Engaging children and young people in research – Literature review.* London: National Evaluation of the Children's Fund. Retrieved from www.ne-cf.org on 13 March 2013.

Coar, L. & Sim, J. (2006). Interviewing one's peers: Methodological issues in a study of health professionals. *Scandinavian Journal of Primary Health Care, 24*, 251–256.

Cocks, A. (2006). The ethical maze: Finding an inclusive path towards gaining children's agreement to research participation. *Childhood, 13*(2), 247–266.

Coles, J. & Mudlay, N. (2010). Staying safe: Strategies for qualitative child abuse researchers. *Child Abuse Review, 19*, 56–69.

Convery, I. & Cox, D. (2012). A review of research ethics in internet-based research. *Practitioner Research in Higher Education, 6*(1), 50–57.

Cook, C. (2011). Email interviewing: Generating data with a vulnerable population. *Journal of Advanced Nursing, 68*(6), 1330–1339.

Corbin, J. & Morse, J. (2003). The unstructured interactive interview: Issues of reciprocity and risks when dealing with sensitive topics. *Qualitative Inquiry, 9*(3), 335–354.

Corden, A. & Sainsbury, R. (2006). Exploring 'quality': Research participants' perspectives on verbatim quotations. *International Journal of Social Research Methodology, 9*(2), 97–110.

Corsaro, W. (2011). *The sociology of childhood* (Third edition). California: Pine Forge Press.

Coyne, I. (2010). Accessing children as research participants: Examining the role of gatekeepers. *Child: Care, Health and Development, 36*(4), 452–454.

Creswell, J. (2003). *Research design: Qualitative, quantitative and mixed methods approaches* (Second edition). London: Sage.

Cresswell, J. (2005). *Writing for academic success: A postgraduate guide.* London: Sage.

Cromby, J. & Nightingale, D. J. (1999). What's wrong with social constructionism? In D. Nightingale, and J. Cromby (eds), *Social constructionist psychology: A critical analysis of theory and practice* (pp. 1–20). Buckingham: Open University Press.

Cunningham, S. (2004). How to … write a paper. *Journal of Orthodontics, 31*, 47–51.

Danby, S., Ewing, L. & Thorpe, K. (2011). The novice researcher: Interviewing young children. *Qualitative Inquiry, 17*(1), 74–84.

Davidson, C. (2009). Transcription: Imperatives for research. *International Journal of Qualitative Research, 8*(2), 35–52.

Davies, B. (2005). Coercion or collaboration? Nurses doing research with people who have severe mental health problems. *Journal of Psychiatric and Mental Health Nursing, 12*, 106–111.

Davies, H., Nutley, S. & Smith, P. (eds) (2000). *What works? Evidence-based policy and practice in public services.* Bristol, UK: The Policy Press.

DeLeeuw, E., Borgers, N. & Smits, A. (2004). Pretesting questionnaires for children and adolescents. In S. Presser, J. Rothgeb, M. Couper, J. Lessler, E. Martin, J. Martin & E. Singer (eds), *Methods for testing and evaluating survey questionnaires* (pp. 409–430). New York: John Wiley.

Department of Health (1999). *Research – What's in it for consumers? Report of the Standing Advisory Committee on consumer involvement in the NHS research and development programme.* London: Department of Health.

Devers, K. (1999). How will we know 'good' qualitative research when we see it? Beginning the dialogue in health services research. *Health Services Research, 34*(5), 1153–1188.

Dickson-Swift, V., James, E., Kippen, S. & Liamputtong, P. (2006). Blurring boundaries in qualitative health research on sensitive topics. *Qualitative Health Research, 16*(6), 853–871.

Dickson-Swift, V., James, E., Kippen, S. & Liamputtong, P. (2008). Risk to researchers in qualitative research on sensitive topics: Issues and strategies. *Qualitative Health Research, 18*(1), 133–144.

Dixon-Woods, M., Angell, E., Ashcroft, R. & Bryman, A. (2007). Written work: The social functions of Research Ethics Committee letters. *Social Science and Medicine, 65*, 792–802.

Dixon-Woods, M., Tarrant, C., Jackson, C., Jones, D. & Kenyon, S. (2011). Providing the results of research to participants: A mixed-method study of the benefits and challenges of a consultative approach. *Clinical Trials, 8*, 330–341.

Drew, P. (2006). When documents 'speak': Documents, language and interaction. In P. Drew, G. Raymond & D. Weinberg (eds), *Talk and interaction in social research methods* (pp. 63–80). London: Sage.

Drew, S., Duncan, R. & Sawyer, S. (2010). Visual storytelling: A beneficial but challenging method for health research with young people. *Qualitative Health Research, 20*(12), 1677–1688.

Driessnack, M. (2006). Draw-and-tell conversations with children about fear. *Qualitative Health Research', 16*, 1414–1435.

DuBois, J. (2008). *Ethics in mental health research: Principles, guidance, and cases.* Oxford: Oxford University Press.

Duffy, M. (2000). The internet as a research and dissemination resource. *Health Promotion International, 15*(4), 349–353.

Dunn, L., Kim, D., Fellows, I. & Palmer, B. (2009). Worth the risk? Relationship of incentives to risk and benefit perceptions and willingness to participate in schizophrenia research. *Schizophrenia Bulletin, 35*(4), 730–737.

Duranti, A. (2007). Transcripts, like shadows on a wall. *Mind, Culture, and Activity, 13*(4), 301–310.

Eastham, L. (2011). Research using blogs for data: Public documents or private musings? *Research in Nursing and Health, 34,* 353–361.

Eder, D. & Corsaro, W. (1999). Ethnographic studies of children and youth: Theoretical and ethical issues. *Journal of Contemporary Ethnography, 28*(5), 520–531.

Edwards, D., Ashmore, M. & Potter, J. (1995). Death and furniture: The rhetoric, politics and theology of bottom line arguments against relativism. *History of the Human Sciences, 8*(2), 25–49.

Edwards, D. & Potter, J. (1992). *Discursive Psychology.* London: Sage.

Elliott, H. (1997). The use of diaries in sociological research on health experience. *Sociological Research Online, 2*(2). Retrieved from www.socresonline.org. uk/2/2/7/.html on 17 March 2013.

Emmel, N., Hughes, K., Greenhalgh, J. & Sales, A. (2007). Accessing socially excluded people: Trust and the gatekeeper in the researcher-participant relationship. *Sociological Research Online, 12*(2). Retrieved from www.socresonline.org. uk/12/2/emmel.html doi: 10.5153/sro.1512 on 19 March 2013.

Etherington, K. (1996). The counsellor as researcher: Boundary issues and critical dilemmas. *British Journal of Guidance and Counselling, 24,* 339–346.

Etherington, K. (2001). Research with ex-clients: A celebration and extension of the therapeutic process. *British Journal of Guidance and Counselling, 29*(1), 5–19.

Etherington, K. (2007). Working with traumatic stories: From transcriber to witness. *International Journal of Social Research Methodology, 10*(2), 85–97.

Evans, A., Elford, J. & Wiggins, D. (2008). Using the internet for qualitative research. In C. Willig & W. Stainton-Rogers (eds), *The Sage handbook of qualitative research in psychology* (pp. 315–333). London: Sage.

Eve, J. (2008). Writing a research proposal: Planning and communicating your research ideas effectively. *Library and Information Research, 32*(102), 18–28.

Eysenbach, G. & Till, J. (2001). Ethical issues in qualitative research on internet communities. *British Medical Journal, 323,* 1103–1105.

Farquhar, C. & Das, R. (1998). Are focus groups suitable for sensitive topics? In R. Barbour & J. Kitzinger (eds), *Developing focus group research: Politics, theory and practice.* Thousand Oaks, CA: Sage.

Faulkner, A. (2004). *The ethics of survivor research: Guidelines for the ethical conduct of research carried out by mental health service users and survivors.* Bristol: Polity Press.

Fernandez, C., Gao, J., Strahlendorf, C., Moghrabi, A., Davis Pentz, R., Barfield, R., Baker, J., Santor, D.,Weijer, C. & Kodish, E. (2009). Providing research results to participants: Attitudes and needs of adolescents and parents of children with cancer. *Journal of Clinical Oncology, 27*(6), 878–883.

Field, M. & Behrman, R. (eds) (2004). *Ethical conduct of clinical research involving children.* Washington: Institute of Medicine, the National Academic Press.

Fink, A. (2005). *Conducting research literature reviews: From the internet to paper* (Second edition). London: Sage.

Finlay, L. (2002). 'Outing' the researcher: The provenance, process, and practice of reflexivity. *Qualitative Health Research*, *12*(4), 531–545.

Finlay, L. (2003). The reflexive journey: Mapping multiple routes. In L. Finlay & B. Gough (eds), *Reflexivity: A practical guide for researchers in health and social sciences* (pp. 3–20). Oxford: Blackwell.

Fisher, C., Hoagwood, L., Boyce, C., Duster, T., Frank, D., Grisso, T., Levine, R., Macklin, R., Spencer, M., Takanishi, R., Trimble, J. & Zayas, L. (2002). Research ethics for mental health science involving ethnic minority children and youths. *American Psychologist*, *57*(12), 1024–1040.

Flewitt, R. (2005). Conducting research with young children: Some ethical considerations. *Early Child Development and Care*, *175*(6), 553–565.

Flynn, N. (2004). *Instant messaging rules: A business guide to managing policies, security, and legal issues for safe IM communication*. Saranac Lake, NY: AMACOM.

Fontes, T. & O'Mahony, M. (2008). In-depth interviewing by Instant Messenger. *Social Research update*, *53*, online. Retrieved from www.soc.surrey.ac.uk/sru on 20 February 2013.

Fox, J., Murray, C. & Warm, A. (2003). Conducting research using web-based questionnaires: Practical, methodological, and ethical considerations. *International Journal of Social Research Methodology*, *6*(2), 167–180.

Francis, J., Johnston, M., Robertson, C., Glidewell, L., Entwistle, V., Eccles, M. & Grimshaw, J. (2010). What is adequate sample size? Operationalising data saturation for theory-based interview studies. *Psychology and Health*, *25*(10), 1229–1245.

Fraser, M. & Fraser, A. (2001). Are people with learning disabilities able to contribute to focus groups on health promotion? *Journal of Advanced Nursing*, *33*(2), 225–233.

Freeman, M. & Mathison, S. (2009). *Researching children's experiences*. New York: The Guildford Press.

Gallacher, L-A. & Gallagher, M. (2008). Methodological immaturity in childhood research? Thinking through 'participatory methods'. *Childhood*, *15*(4), 499–516.

Gallagher, M. (2008). 'Power is not an evil': Rethinking power in participatory methods. *Children's Geographies*, *6*(2), 137–150.

Gans, J. & Brindis, C. (1995). Choice of research setting in understanding adolescent health problems. *Journal of Adolescent Health*, *17*, 306–313.

Garfinkel, H. (1967). *Studies in ethnomethodology*. Malden, USA: Blackwell.

Garth, B. & Aroni, R. (2003). 'I value what you have to say'. Seeking the perspective of children with a disability, not just their parents. *Disability and Society*, *18*(5), 561–576.

Gaskell, G. (2000). Individual and group interviewing. In M. Bauer & G. Gaskell (eds), *Qualitative researching with text, image and sound* (pp. 38–56). London: Sage.

Geluda, K., Bisaglia, J., Moreira, V., Maldonado, B. M., Cunha, A. & Trajman, A. (2005). Third-party informed consent in research with adolescents: The good, the bad and the ugly. *Social Science and Medicine*, *61*, 985–988.

Gibbs, G., Friese, S. & Mangabeira, W. (2002). The use of new technology in qualitative research. *Forum: Qualitative Social Research*, *3*(2), online. Retrieved from www. qualitative-research.net/index.php/fqs/article/view/847/1840 on 25 March 2013.

Gilgun, J. (2005). 'Grab' and good science: Writing up the results of qualitative research. *Qualitative Health Research*, *15*(2), 256–262.

Giordano, J., O'Reilly, M., Taylor, H. & Dogra, N. (2007). Confidentiality and autonomy: The challenge(s) of offering research participants a choice of disclosing their identity. *Qualitative Health Research, 17*(2), 264–275.

Goering, P., Boydell, K. & Pignatiello, A. (2008). The relevance of qualitative research for clinical programs in psychiatry. *Canadian Journal of Psychiatry, 53*, 145–151.

Goldblatt, H., Karnieli-Miller, O. & Neumann, M. (2011). Sharing qualitative research findings with participants: Study experiences of methodological and ethical dilemmas. *Patient Education and Counseling, 82*, 389–395.

Gollop, M. (2000). Interviewing children: A research perspective. In A. Smith, N. Taylor & M. Gollop (eds), *Children's voices: Research, policy and practice* (pp. 18–34). New Zealand: Longman.

Goodare, H. & Lockwood, S. (1999). Involving patients in clinical research. *British Medical Journal, 319*, 724–725.

Gordner, C. & Burkett, L. (2012). Writing a poster abstract: Guidelines for success. *PENS Reporter, 3*, 5–6.

Gough, B. (2003). Deconstructing reflexivity. In L. Finlay & B. Gough (eds), *Reflexivity: A practical guide for researchers in health and social sciences* (pp. 21–36). Oxford: Blackwell.

Grady, C. (2005). Payment of clinical research subjects. *The Journal of Clinical Investigation, 115* (7), 1681–1687.

Grant, J. & Luxford, Y. (2009). Video: A decolonising strategy for intercultural communication in child and family health within ethnographic research. *International Journal of Multiple Research Approaches, 3*, 218–232.

Green, A., Rafaeli, E., Bolger, N., Shrout, P. & Reis, H. (2006). Paper or plastic? Data equivalence in paper and electronic diaries. *Psychological Methods, 11*(1), 87–105.

Green, J., Franquiz, M. & Dixon, C. (1997). The myth of the objective transcript: Transcribing as a situated act. *TESOL Quarterly, 31*(1), 172–176.

Greenhalgh, T. (1997). How to read a paper: Getting your bearings (deciding what the paper is about). *British Medical Journal, 315*, 243–246.

Greenhalgh, T. & Taylor, R. (1997). How to read a paper: Papers that go beyond numbers (qualitative research). *British Medical Journal, 315*, 740–743.

Gregory, D., Russell, C. & Phillips, L. (1997). Beyond textual perfection: Transcribers as vulnerable persons. *Qualitative Health Research, 7*(2), 294–300.

Greig, A., Taylor, J. & MacKay, T. (2007). *Doing research with children* (Second edition). London: Sage.

Grimandi, S. (2007). Commentary: Some reflections on the use of video recordings. *Infant Observation, 10*(10), 89–90.

Grimshaw, A. (1982). Sound-image data records for research on social interaction: Some questions and answers. *Sociological Methods and Research, 11*, 121–144.

Grol, R. & Grimshaw, J. (2003). From best evidence to best practice: Effective implementation of change in patients' care. *Lancet, 362*, 1225–1230.

Guba, E. G. & Lincoln, Y. (2004). Competing paradigms in qualitative research: Theories and issues. In S. Hesse-Biber & P. Leavy (eds), *Approaches to qualitative research: A reader on theory and practice* (pp. 17–38). Oxford: Oxford University Press.

Halcomb, E. & Davidson, P. (2006). Is verbatim transcription of interview data always necessary? *Applied Nursing Research, 19*, 38–42.

Halliwell, E., Main, L. & Richardson, C. (2007). *The fundamental facts: The latest facts and figures on mental health*. The Mental Health Foundation.

Hamilton, R. & Bowers, B. (2006). Internet recruitment and e-mail interviews in qualitative studies. *Qualitative Health Research, 16*(6), 821–835.

Hammersley, M. (1985). Ethnography: What it is and what it offers. In S. Hegarty & P. Evans, (eds), *Research and evaluation methods in special education* (pp. 152–163). *Philadelphia*: NFER-Nelson.

Hammersley, M. (2010). Reproducing or constructing? Some questions about transcription in social research. *Qualitative Research, 10*(5), 553–569.

Hamo, M., Blum-Kulka, S. & Hacohen, G. (2004). From observation to transcription and back: Theory, practice, and interpretation in the analysis of children's naturally occurring discourse. *Research on Language and Social Interaction, 37*(1), 71–92.

Happell, B. (2007). Hitting the target! A no tears approach to writing an abstract for a conference presentation. *International Journal of Mental Health Nursing, 16*, 477–452.

Happell, B. (2009). Presenting with precision: Preparing and delivering a polished conference presentation. *Nurse Researcher, 16*(3), 45–55.

Harden, J., Scott, S., Backett-Milburn, K. & Jackson, S. (2000). Can't talk, won't talk: Methodological issues in researching children. *Sociological Research Online 5*. Retrieved from www.socresonline.org.uk/5/2/harden.html on 16 January 2013.

Hart, N. & Crawford-Wright, A. (1999). Research as therapy, therapy as research: Ethical dilemmas in new-paradigm research. *British Journal of Guidance & Counselling, 27*(2), 205–214.

Heath, C. (2004). Analysing face-to-face interaction: Video, the visual and material. In D. Silverman (ed.), *Qualitative research: Theory, method and practice* (Second edition) (pp. 266–282). London: Sage.

Heath, S., Charles, V., Crow, G. & Wiles, R. (2004). Informed consent, gatekeepers & go-betweens. Paper presented at *The Ethics & Social Relations of Research* conference (Sixth International Conference on Social Science Methodology): Amsterdam.

Heath, S., Charles, V., Crow, G. & Wiles, R. (2007). Informed consent, gatekeepers and go-betweens: Negotiating consent in child and youth-oriented institutions. *British Educational Research Journal, 33* (3), 403–417.

Hepburn, A. & Bolden, G. (2013). The conversation analytic approach to transcription. In T. Stivers & J. Sidnell (eds), *The Blackwell handbook of conversation analysis* (pp. 57–76). Oxford: Blackwell.

Heptinstall, E. (2000). Gaining access to looked after children for research purposes: Lessons learned. *British Journal of Social Work, 30*, 867–872.

Herring, A. (1996). Linguistic and critical analysis of computer-mediated communication: Some ethical and scholarly considerations. *The Information Society, 12*(2), 153–168.

Hewson, C., Laurent, D. & Vogel, C. (1996). Proper methodologies for psychological and sociological studies conducted via the internet. *Behaviour Research Methods, Instruments and Computers, 28*, 186–191.

Hill, M. (1997). Participatory research with children. *Child and Family Social Work, 2*, 171–183.

Hinchcliffe, V. & Gavin, H. (2009). Social and virtual networks: Evaluating synchronous online interviewing using instant messenger. *The Qualitative Report, 14*(2), 318–340.

Hoagwood, K., Burns, B., Kiser, L., Ringeisem, H. & Schoenwald, S. (2001). Evidence-based practice in child and adolescent mental health services. *Psychiatric Services*, *52*(9), 1179–1189.

Hoagwood, K., Jensen, P. & Fisher, C. (1996). Toward a science of ethics in research on child and adolescent mental disorders. In K. Hoagwood, P. Jensen & C. Fisher (eds), *Ethical issues in mental health research with children and adolescents* (pp. 3–14). New Jersey: Lawrence Earlbaum Associates.

Holmes, D., Hodgson, P., Nishmura, R. & Simari, R. (2009). Manuscript preparation and publication. *Circulation*, *120*, 906–913.

Holmes, S. (2009). Methodological and ethical considerations in designing an internet study of quality of life. *A discussion paper, International Journal of Nursing Studies*, *46*, 394–405.

Holoday, B. & Turner-Henson, A. (1989). Response effects in surveys with school-age children. *Nursing Research*, *38*, 248–250.

Holt, L. (2004). The 'voices' children: De-centring empowering research relations. *Children's Geographies*, *2*(1), 13–27.

Hookway, N. (2008). Entering the blogosphere: Some strategies for using blogs in social research. *Qualitative Research*, *8*, 91–113.

Hoppe, M., Wells, E., Morrison, D., Gillmore, M. & Wilsdon, A. (1995). Using focus groups to discuss sensitive topics with children. *Evaluation Review*, *19*(1), 102–114.

Horstman, M., Aldiss, S., Richardson, A. & Gibson, F. (2008). Methodological issues when using the draw and write technique with children aged 6–12 years. *Qualitative Health Research*, *18*(7), 1001–1011.

Hubbard, G., Backett-Milburn, K. & Kemmer, D. (2001). Working with emotion: Issues for the researcher in fieldwork and teamwork. *International Journal of Social Research Methodology*, *4*(2), 119–137.

Hudson, J. & Bruckman, A. (2004). 'Go away'? Participant objections to being studied and the ethics of chatroom research. *The Information Society*, *20*(2), 127–139.

Hunt, N. & McHale, S. (2007). A practical guide to the e-mail interview. *Qualitative Health Research*, *17*, 1415–1421.

Hunter, D. & Pierscionek, B. (2007). Children, Gillick competency and consent for involvement in research. *Journal of Medical Ethics*, *33*, 659–662.

Hutchby, I. (2002). Resisting the incitement to talk in child counselling: Aspects of the utterance 'I don't know'. *Discourse Studies*, *4*(2), 147–168.

Hutchby, I. & Wooffitt, R. (2008). *Conversation analysis* (Second edition). Oxford: Blackwell.

Irwin, L. & Johnson, J. (2005). Interviewing young children: Explicating our practices and dilemmas. *Qualitative Health Research*, *15*, 821–831

Ison, N. (2009). Having their say: Email interviews for research data collection with people who have verbal communication impairment. *International Journal of Social Research Methodology*, *12*(2), 161–172.

Israel, B., Schulz, A., Parker, E. & Becker, A. (1998). Review of community-based research: Assessing partnership approaches to improve public health. *Annual Review Public Health*, *19*, 173–202.

Jacelon, C. & Imperio, K. (2005). Participant diaries as a source of data in research with older adults. *Qualitative Health Research*, *15*(7), 991–997.

James, A. (2001). Ethnography in the study of children and childhood. In P. Atkinson, A. Coffey, S. Delamont, J. Lofland & L. Lofland (eds), *Handbook of ethnography* (pp. 256–257). London: Sage.

James, N., and Busher, H. (2006). Credibility, authenticity and voice: Dilemmas in online interviewing. *Qualitative Research, 6*(3), 403–420.

Jefferson, G. (2004). Glossary of transcript symbols with an introduction. In G. H. Lerner (ed.), *Conversation analysis: Studies from the first generation* (pp. 13–31). Amsterdam: John Benjamins.

Joffe, H. & Yardley, L. (2004) Content and thematic analysis. In D. Marks & L. Yardley (eds), *Research methods for clinical and health psychology* (pp. 56–68). London: Sage.

Johns, C. & Freshwater, D. (1998). *Transforming nursing through reflective practice.* London: Blackwell Science.

Johnson, B. & Macleod-Clark, J. (2003). Collecting sensitive data: The impact on researchers. *Qualitative Health Research, 13*(3), 421–434.

Johnson, T. (2008). Tips on how to write a paper. *Journal American Academy Dermatology, 59*(6), 1064–1069.

Jordhoy, M., Kaasa,S., Fayers, P., Overness, T., Underland, G. & Ahlner-Elmqvist, M. (1999). Challenges in palliative care research; recruitment, attrition and compliance: Experience from a randomized controlled trial. *Palliative Medicine, 13,* 299–310.

Jowett, A., Peel, E. & Shaw, R. (2011). Online interviewing in psychology: Reflections on the process. *Qualitative Research in Psychology, 8,* 354–369.

Kaiser, K. (2009). Protecting respondent confidentiality in qualitative research. *Qualitative Health Research, 19*(11), 1632–1641.

Karchmer, R. (2001). The journey ahead: Thirteen teachers report how the internet influences literacy and literacy instruction in their K-12 classrooms. *Reading Research Quarterly, 36*(4), 442–466.

Kearney, M. (2001). Levels and applications of qualitative research evidence. *Research in Nursing and Health, 24,* 145–153.

Keen, S. & Todres, L. (2007). Strategies for disseminating qualitative research findings: Three exemplars. *Forum: Qualitative Social Research, 8*(3), *Art 17,* Retrieved from www.qualitative-research.net/fqs on 11 April 2013.

Kerrison, S., McNally, N. & Pollock, A. (2003). United Kingdom research governance strategy. *British Medical Journal, 327,* 553–556.

Kidd, J. & Finlayson, M. (2006). Navigating unchartered water: Research ethics and emotional engagement in human inquiry. *Journal of Psychiatric and Mental Health Nursing, 13,* 423–428.

King, N. & Churchill, L. (2000). Ethical principles guiding research on child and adolescent subjects. *Journal of Interpersonal Violence, 12*(6), 710–724.

Kitchener, K. (1988). Dual role relationships – what makes them so problematic? *Journal of Counseling and Development, 67,* 217–221.

Kitzinger, J. (1994). The methodology of focus groups: The importance of interaction between research participants. *Sociology of Health and Illness, 16,* 103–121.

Knupfer, A. (1996). Ethnographic studies of children: The difficulties of entry, rapport, and presentation of their worlds. *Qualitative Studies in Education, 9*(2), 135–149.

Koo, M. & Skinner, H. (2005). Challenges of internet recruitment: A case study with disappointing results. *Journal of Med Internet Research, 7*(1), e6.

Kuhn, T. (1962). *The structure of scientific revolutions*. Chicago: University of Chicago Press.

Kuper, A., Lingard, L. & Levinson, W. (2008). Critically appraising qualitative research. *British Medical Journal, 337*, 687–689.

Kuper, A., Reeves, S. & Levinson, W. (2008). An Introduction to reading and appraising qualitative research. *British Medical Journal, 337*, 404–407.

Kvale, S. (2006). Dominance through interviews and dialogues. *Qualitative Inquiry, 12*(3), 480–500.

Kvale, S. & Brinkman, S. (2009). *Interviewing: Learning the craft of qualitative research interviewing* (Second edition). London: Sage.

Lalor, J., Begley, C. & Devane, D. (2006). Exploring painful experiences: Impact of emotional narratives on members of a qualitative research team. *Journal of Advanced Nursing, 56*(6), 607–616.

Lapadat, J. (2000). Problematizing transcription: Purpose, paradigm and quality. *International Journal of Social Research Methodology, 3*(3), 203–219.

Lapadat, J. & Lindsay, A. (1999). Transcription in research and practice: From standardization of technique to interpretive positioning. *Qualitative Inquiry, 5*(1), 64–86.

LeCompte, M. and Goetz, J. (1982). Problems of reliability and validity in ethnographic research. *Review of Educational Research, 52*(1), 31–60.

Lenhart, A. & Madden, M. (2007). *Teens, privacy and online social networks: How teens manage their online identities and personal information in the age of MySpace*. Washington: DC: Pew Internet and American Life Project.

Levine, C., Faden, R., Grady, C., Hammerschmidt, D., Eckenwiler, L. & Sugarman, J. (2004). The limitations of 'vulnerability' as a protection for human research participants. *The American Journal of Bioethics, 4*(3), 44–49.

Lewis, A. (1992). Group child interviews as a research tool. *British Educational Research Journal, 18*(4), 413–421.

Lewis, K., Kaufman, J., Gonzalez, M., Wimmer, A. & Christakis, N. (2008). Tastes, ties, and time: A new social network dataset using Facebook.com. *Social Networks, 30*, 330–342.

Liamputtong, P. (2007). *Researching the vulnerable: A guide to sensitive research methods*. Thousand Oaks, CA: Sage.

Liebling, A. (1999). Doing research in prison: Breaking the silence? *Theoretical Criminology, 3*(2), 147–173.

Liegghio, M., Nelson, G. & Evans, S. (2010). Partnering with children diagnosed with mental health issues: Contributions of a sociology of childhood perspective of participatory action research. *American Journal of Psychology, 46*, 84–99.

Lincoln, Y. & Guba, E. (1985). *Naturalistic inquiry*. Thousand Oaks, CA: Sage.

Livingstone, S. (2003). Children's use of the internet: Reflections on the emerging research agenda. *New Media & Society, 5*(2), 147–166.

Lowcay, B. & McIntyre, E. (2005). Research posters – the way to display. *British Medical Journal*, December, 251–252.

Lucas, K. (2010). A waste of time? The value and promise of researcher completed qualitative data transcribing. *Northeastern Educational Research Association Conference Proceedings, paper 24*. Retrieved from http://digitalcommons.uconn.edu/nera_2010/24 on 5 May 2012.

MacDonald, K. (2008). Dealing with chaos and complexity: The reality of interviewing children and families in their own homes. *Journal of Clinical Nursing, 17*(23), 3123–3130.

Mackrill, T. (2008). Solicited diary studies of psychotherapy in qualitative research – pros and cons. *European Journal of Psychotherapy and Counselling, 10*(1), 5–18.

Magnuson, S., Wilcoxon, S.A. & Norem, K. (2000). A profile of lousy supervision: Experienced counselors' perspectives. *Counselor Education and Supervision, 39*, 189–202.

Mander, R. (1992). Seeking approval for research access: The gatekeeper's role in facilitating a study of the care of the relinquishing mother. *Journal of Advanced Nursing, 17*, 1460–1464.

Markham, M. (2006). Providing research participants with findings from completed cancer-related clinical trials: Not quite as simple as it sounds. *Cancer, 106*, 1421–1424.

Marshall, M. (1996). Sampling for qualitative research. *Family Practice, 13*(6), 522–525.

Mauthner, M. (1997). Methodological aspects of collecting data from children; lessons from three research projects. *Children and Society, 11*, 16–28.

Mayer, M. & Till, J. (1996). The internet: A modern Pandora's box? *Qualitative Life Research, 5*, 568–571.

Mays, N. & Pope, C. (2000). Quality in qualitative health research. In C. Pope & N. Mays (eds), *Qualitative research in health care* (pp. 89–102). London: BMJ Books.

McCormick, L., Crawford, M., Anderson, R., Gittelsohn, J., Kingsley, B. & Upson, D. (1999). Recruiting adolescents into qualitative tobacco research studies: Experiences and lessons learned. *Journal of School Health, 69*(3), 95–99.

McCosker, H. Barnard, A. & Gerber, R. (2001). Undertaking sensitive research: Issues and strategies for meeting the safety needs of all participants. *Forum: Qualitative Social Research, 2*(1). Retrieved from www.qualitative-research.net/index.php/fqs/article/view/983 on 14 May 2014.

McNeill, P. (1997). Paying people to participate in research: Why not? A response to Wilkinson and Moore. *Bioethics, 11*(5), 390–396.

McPherson, A. (2010). Involving children: Why it matters. In S. Redsell & A. Hastings (eds), *Listening to children and young people in healthcare consultations* (pp. 15–30). Oxford: Radcliffe Publishing.

McWhinney, I., Bass, M. & Donner, A. (1994). Evaluation of a palliative care service: Problems and pitfalls. *British Medical Journal, 309*, 1340–1342.

Meho, L. (2006). E-mail interviewing in qualitative research: A methodological discussion. *Journal of the American Society for Information Science and Technology, 57*(10), 1284–1295.

Melo-Martin, I. & Ho, A. (2008). Beyond informed consent: The therapeutic misconception and trust. *Journal of Medical Ethics, 34*, 202–205.

Meltzer, D., Fryers, T. & Jenkins, R. (eds) (2004). *Social inequalities and the distribution of the common mental health disorders*. Hove: Psychology Press.

Mental Health Foundation (1999). What is mental capacity? Retrieved from www.amcat.org.uk/what_is_mental_capacity/ on 20 November 2012.

Merriam, S. (2002). Assessing and evaluating qualitative research. In S. Merriam et al. (eds), *Assessing and evaluating qualitative research in practice* (pp. 18–33). San Francisco: Jossey-Bass.

Miles, B. (2006). Moving out of the dark ages: An argument for the use of digital video in social work research. *Journal of Technology in Human Services. 24*(2/3), 181–196.

Mondada, L. (2007). Commentary: Transcript variations and the indexicality of transcribing practices. *Discourse Studies*, *9*(6), 809–821.

Moreno, M., Fost, N. & Christakis, D. (2008). Research ethics in the MySpace era. *Pediatrics*, *121*(1), 157–161.

Moreno, M., Grant, A., Kacvinsky, L., Moreno, P. & Fleming, M. (2012). Older adolescents' views regarding participation in Facebook research. *Journal of Adolescent Health*, *51*(5), 439–444.

Morgan, A. (2010). Discourse analysis: An overview for the neophyte researcher. *Journal of Health and Social Care Improvement*, *May*, 1–7.

Morgan, M., Gibbs, A., Maxwell, K. & Britten, N. (2002). Hearing children's voices: Methodological issues in conducting focus groups with children aged 7–11 years. *Qualitative Research*, *2*(1), 5–20.

Morrow, V. & Richards, M. (1996). The ethics of social research with children: An overview. *Children and Society*, *10*, 90–105.

Munford, R. & Sanders, J. (2004). Recruiting diverse groups of young people to research: Agency and empowerment in the consent process. *Qualitative Social Work*, *3*(4), 469–482.

Murray, R. (2006). *How to write a thesis* (Second edition). Berkshire: Open University Press.

Nadin, S. & Cassell, C. (2006). The use of a research diary as a tool for reflexive practice: Some reflections from management research. *Qualitative Research in Accounting and Management*, *3*(3), 208–217.

Nightingale, D. & Cromby, J. (eds) (1999). *Social constructionist psychology: A critical analysis of theory and practice*. Buckingham: Open University Press.

Nikander, P. (2008). Working with transcripts and translated data. *Qualitative Research in Psychology*, *5*, 225–231.

Nolan, M. & Grant, G. (1993). Service evaluation: Time to open both eyes. *Journal of Advanced Nursing*, *18*, 1434–1442.

Norman, K., Friedman, Z., Norman, K. & Stevenson, R. (2001). Navigational issues in the design of on-line self-administered questionnaires. *Behaviour and Information Technology*, *20*(1), 37–45.

Nosek, B., Banaji, M. & Greenwald, A. (2002). E-Research: Ethics, security, design, and control in psychological research on the internet. *Journal of Social Issues*, *58*(1), 161–176.

Ochs, E. (1979). Transcription as theory. In E. Ochs & B. Schiefflin (eds), *Developmental Pragmatics* (pp. 43–72). New York: Academic Press.

O'Connor, H. & Madge, C. (2001). Cyber-mothers: Online synchronous interviewing using conferencing software. *Sociological Research Online*, *5*(4). Retrieved from www.socresonline.org.uk/5/4/oconnor.html on 25 March 2013.

Oeye, C., Bjelland, A. & Skorpen, A. (2007). Doing participant observation in a psychiatric hospital – research ethics resumed. *Social Science and Medicine*, *65*, 2296–2306.

Oliver, P. (2010). *The student's guide to research ethics* (Second edition). Berkshire: Open University Press.

Onwuegbuzie, A. & Leech, N. (2007). A call for qualitative power analyses. *Quality & Quantity: An International Journal of Methodology*, *41*, 105–121.

Opdenakker, R. (2006). Advantages and disadvantages of four interview techniques in qualitative research. *Forum Qualitative Sozialforschung/Forum: Qualitative*

Social Research, 7(4), online. Retrieved from www.qualitative-research.net/index. php/fqs/rt/printerfriendly/175/391 on 18 March 2013.

O'Reilly, M. (2005a). Active noising: The use of noises in talk, the case of onomato-poeia, abstract sounds and the functions they serve in therapy. *TEXT* 25(6), 745–761.

O'Reilly, M. (2005b). 'Disabling essentialism': Accountability in family therapy: Issues of disability, complaints and child abuse. Unpublished PhD thesis, Loughborough University.

O'Reilly, M. (2006). Should children be seen and not heard? An examination of how children's interruptions are treated in family therapy. *Discourse Studies*. 8(4), 549–566.

O'Reilly, M., Cook, L. & Karim, K. (2012). Complementary or controversial care? The opinions of professionals on complementary and alternative interventions for Autistic Spectrum Disorder. *Clinical Child Psychology and Psychiatry*, e-pub = doi: 10.1177/1359104511435340.

O'Reilly, M., Dixon-Woods, M., Angell, E., Ashcroft, R. & Bryman, A. (2009). Doing accountability: A discourse analysis of research ethics committee letters. *Sociology of Health and Illness*, 31(2), 246–291.

O'Reilly, M., Karim, K., Taylor, H. & Dogra, N. (2012). Parent and child views on anonymity: 'I've got nothing to hide'. *International Journal of Social Research Methodology*, 15(3), 211–224.

O'Reilly, M. & Parker, N. (2013a). Unsatisfactory saturation': A critical exploration of the notion of saturated sample sizes in qualitative research. *Qualitative Research*, 13(2), 190–197.

O'Reilly, M. & Parker, N. (2013b). 'You can take a horse to water but you can't make it drink': Exploring children's engagement and resistance in family therapy. *Contemporary Family Therapy*, 35(3), 491–507.

O'Reilly, M., Parker, N. & Hutchby, I. (2011). Ongoing processes of managing consent: The empirical ethics of using video-recording in clinical practice and research. *Clinical Ethics*, 6, 179–185.

O'Reilly, M., Ronzoni, P. & Dogra, N. (2013). *Research with children: Theory and practice*. London: Sage.

O'Reilly, M., Taylor, H. & Vostanis, P. (2009). 'Nuts, schiz, psycho': An exploration of young homeless people's perceptions and dilemmas of defining mental health. *Social Science and Medicine*, 68, 1737–1744.

Pantell, R., Stewart, T., Dias, J., Wells, P. & Ross, W. (1982). Physician communication with children and parents. *Pediatrics*, 70(3), 396–402.

Parker, N. & O'Reilly, M. (2012). 'Gossiping' as a social action in family therapy: The pseudo-absence and pseudo-presence of children. *Discourse Studies*, 14(4), 1–19.

Parker, N. & O'Reilly, M. (2013) 'We are alone in the house': A case study addressing researcher safety and risk. *Qualitative Research in Psychology*, doi: 10.1080/14780887.2011.64726.

Parry, G. (1996). Writing a research report. In G. Parry & F. Watts, *Behavioural and mental health research: A handbook of skills and methods* (Second edition) (pp. 137–156). Hove, UK: Earlbaum.

Pascale, C-M. (2011). *Cartographies of knowledge: Exploring qualitative epistemologies*. Thousand Oaks, CA: Sage.

Paterson, B., Gregory, D. & Thorne, S. (1999). A protocol for researcher safety. *Qualitative Health Research, 9*(2), 259–269.

Patton, M. (1990). *Qualitative evaluation and research methods* (Second edition). Thousand Oaks, CA: Sage.

Paul, M., Newns, K. & Creedy, K. (2006). Some ethical issues that arise from working with families in the National Health Service. *Clinical Ethics, 1,* 76–81.

Paulus, T., Lester, J. N. & Dempster, P. (2014). *Digital tools for qualitative research.* London: Sage.

Pearlman, L. & Saakvitne, K. (1995). *Trauma and the therapist: Counter-transference and vicarious traumatisation in psychotherapy with incest survivors.* London: Norton.

Perakyla, A. (2004). Reliability and validity in research based on naturally occurring social interaction. In D. Silverman (ed.), *Qualitative research: Theory, method and practice* (Second edition) (pp. 283–304). London: Sage.

Perakyla, A. (2006). Observation, video and ethnography: Case studies in AIDS counselling and greetings. In P. Drew, G. Raymond & D. Weinberg (eds), *Talk and Interaction in Social Research Methods* (pp. 81–96). London: Sage.

Peters, S. (2010). Qualitative research methods in mental health. *Evidence Based Mental Health, 13*(2), 35–40.

Pierce, M. (1998). Doing research in general practice: Advice for the uninitiated. *Diabetic Medicine, 15* (Suppl. 3), S25–S28.

Piercy, H. & Hargate, M. (2004). Social research on the under-16s: A consideration of the issues from a UK perspective. *Journal of Child Health Care, 8*(4), 253–263.

Plowman, L. & Stephen, C. (2008). The big picture? Video and the representation of interaction. *British Educational Research Journal, 34*(4), 541–565.

Pomerantz, A. & Fehr, B. J. (1997). Conversation analysis: An approach to the study of social action as sense making practices. In T. van Dijk (ed.), *Discourse as social interaction* (pp. 64–91). London: Sage.

Potter, J. (1996). *Representing reality: Discourse, rhetoric and social construction.* London: Sage.

Potter, J. (2002). Two kinds of natural. *Discourse Studies. 4*(4), 539–542.

Potter, J. & Hepburn, A. (2005). Qualitative interviews in psychology: Problems and possibilities. *Qualitative Research in Psychology, 2,* 1–27.

Potter, J. & Wetherell, M. (1987). *Discourse and social psychology.* London: Sage.

Powell, R., Single, H. & Lloyd, K. (1996). Focus groups in mental health research: Enhancing the validity of user and provider questionnaires. *International Journal of Social Psychiatry, 42*(3), 193–206.

Punch, K. (2000). *Developing effective research proposals.* London: Sage.

Punch, S. (2002). Research with children: The same or different from research with adults? *Childhood, 9*(3), 321–341.

Punch, S. (2007). 'I felt they were ganging up on me': Interviewing siblings at home. *Children's geographies, 5*(3), 219–234.

Radden, J. (2002). Psychiatric ethics. *Bioethics, 16*(5), 397–411.

Ranse, J. & Hayes, C. (2009). A novice's guide to preparing and presenting an oral presentation at a scientific conference. *Journal of Emergency Primary Health Care, 7*(1), article 5, available at: http://ro.ecu.edu.au/jephc/vol7/iss1/5 on 11 April 2013.

Rauktis, M., Fiedler, K. & Wood, J. (1998). Focus groups, program evaluation and the mentally ill: A case study. *Journal of Health and Social Policy, 10*(2), 75–92.

Rawson, R., McCann, M., Huber, A., Marinelli-Casey, P. & Williams, L. (2000). Moving research into community settings in the CSAT Methampehetamine treatment project: The coordinating center perspective. *Journal of Psychoactive Drugs, 32*(2), 201–208.

Rew, L., Taylor-Seehafer, M. & Thomas, N. (2000). Without parental consent: Conducting research with homeless adolescents. *Journal of the Society of Pediatric Nurses, 5*(3), 131–138.

Rice, M., Bunker, K., Kang, D., Howell, C. & Weaver, M. (2007). Accessing and recruiting children for research in schools. *Western Journal of Nursing Research, 29*(4), 501–514.

Richards, H. & Emslie, C. (2000). The 'doctor' or the 'girl from the University'? Considering the influence of professional roles on qualitative interviewing. *Family Practice, 17*(10), 71–75.

Richards, H. & Schwartz, L. (2002). Ethics of qualitative research: Are there special issues for health services research? *Family Practice, 19*, 135–139.

Richardson, A. (1994). The health diary: An examination of its use as a data collection method. *Journal of Advanced Nursing, 19*, 782–791.

Riessman, C. K. (2005). Narrative analysis. In N. Kelly, C. Horrocks, K. Milnes, B. Roberts & D. Robinson (eds), *Narrative, memory and everyday life* (pp. 1–7). Huddersfield: University of Huddersfield.

Rishel, C. (2007). Evidence-based prevention practice in mental health: What is it and how do we get there? *American Journal of Orthopsychiatry, 77*(1), 153–164.

Roberts, F. & Robinson, J. (2004). Interobserver agreement on first-stage conversation analytic transcription. *Health Communication Research, 30*(3), 376–410.

Robson, C. (2011). *Real world research* (Third edition). Oxford: Blackwell.

Roszkowski, M. & Bean, A. (1990). Believe it or not! Longer questionnaires have lower response rates. *Journal of Business and Psychology, 4*(4), 495–509.

Roulston, K. (2006). Close encounters of the 'CA' kind: A review of literature analysing talk in research interviews. *Qualitative Research, 6*(4), 515–534.

Roulston, K. (2010). Considering quality in qualitative interviewing. *Qualitative Research, 10*(2), 199–228.

Rowan, M. (1997). Qualitative research articles: Information for authors and peer reviewers. *Canadian Medical Association Journal, 157*, 1442–1446.

Roy-Chowdhury, S. (2003). Knowing the unknowable: What constitutes evidence in family therapy? *Journal of Family Therapy, 25*, 64–85.

Rycroft-Malone, J., Harvey, G., Seers, K., Kitson, A., McCormack, B. & Titchen, A. (2004). An exploration of the factors that influence the implementation of evidence into practice. *Issues in Clinical Nursing, 13*, 913–924.

Sacks, H., Schegloff, E.A. & Jefferson, G. (1974). A simplest systematics for the organization of turn-taking for conversation. *Language, 50*(4), 696–735.

Sampson, H. (2004). Navigating the waves: The usefulness of a pilot in qualitative research. *Qualitative Research, 4*(3), 383–402.

Sampson. H., Bloor, M. & Fincham, B. (2008). A price worth paying? Considering the 'cost' of reflexive research methods and the influence of feminist ways of 'doing'. *Sociology, 42*(5), 919–933.

Sandelowski, M. (2004). Using qualitative research. *Qualitative Health Research*, *14*(10), 1366–1386.

Sandelowski, M. & Barroso, J. (2002). Reading qualitative studies. *International Journal of Qualitative Methods*, *1*(1), article 5. Retrieved from https://ejournals.library.ualberta.ca/index.php/IJQM/article/view/4521/3651 on 11 January 2013.

Sandelowski, M. & Barroso, J. (2003). Writing the proposal for a qualitative research methodology project. *Qualitative Health Research*, *13*(6), 781–820.

Schmidt, W. (1997). World-wide web survey research: Benefits, potential problems, and solutions. *Behaviour Research Methods, Instruments & Computers*, *29*, 274–279.

Schön, D. (1983). *The reflective practitioner.* New York: Basic Books.

Scott, J., Wishart, J. & Bowyer, D. (2006). Do current consent and confidentiality requirements impede or enhance research with children with learning disabilities? *Disability and Society*, *21*(3), 273–287.

Sharpe, D. & Baker, D. (2007). Financial issues associated with having a child with autism. *Journal of Family and Economic Issues*, *28*, 247–264.

Sharples, M., Graber, R., Harrison, C. & Logan, K. (2009). E-safety and Web 2.0 for children aged 11–16. *Journal of Computer Assisted Learning*, *25*, 70–84.

Shaw, I. (2008). Ethics and the practice of qualitative research. *Qualitative Social Work*, *7*(4), 400–414.

Sieber, J. (1992). *Planning ethically responsible research: A guide for students and internal review boards.* Newbury Park: Sage.

Silverman, D. (2006). *Interpreting qualitative data: Methods for analysing talk, text and interaction* (Third edition). London: Sage.

Silverman, D. (2009). *Doing qualitative research* (Third edition). London: Sage.

Sinding, C. & Aronson, J. (2003). Exposing failures, unsettling accommodations: Tensions in interview practice. *Qualitative Research*, *3*(1), 95–117.

Singh, I. & Keenan, S. (2010). The challenges and opportunities of qualitative health research with children. In I. Bourgeault, R. Dingwall & R. DeVries (eds), *The Sage handbook of qualitative methods in health research* (pp. 696–713). London: Sage.

Skukauskaite, A. (2012). Transparency in transcribing: Making visible theoretical bases impacting knowledge construction from open-ended interview records. *Forum: Qualitative Social Research*, *13*(1). Retrieved from www.qualitative-research.net/index.php/fqs/article/view/1532 on 14 May 2014.

Small, S. (2005). Bridging research and practice in the family and human sciences. *Family Relations*, *54*, 320–334.

Smith, B. (1999). Ethical and methodologic benefits of using a reflexive journal in hermeneutic-phenomenologic research. *Journal of Nursing Scholarship*, *31*(4), 359–363.

Smith, J. A. (2004). Reflecting on the development of interpretative phenomenological analysis and its contribution to qualitative research in psychology. *Qualitative Research in Psychology*, *1*, 39–54.

Social Research Association (2005). 'Staying safe: A code of practice for the safety of social researchers'. Retrieved from www.the-sra.org.uk on 18 October 2012.

Sparrman, A. (2005). Video recording as interaction: Participant observation of children's everyday life. *Qualitative Research in Psychology*, *2*, 241–255.

Speer, S. (2002). 'Natural' and 'contrived' data: A sustainable distinction? *Discourse Studies*, *4*(4), 511–525.

Speer, S. & Hutchby, I. (2003). From ethics to analytics: Aspects of participants' orientations to the presence and relevance of recording devices. *Sociology*, *37*(2), 315–337.

Spencer, L., Ritchie, J., Lewis, J. & Dillon, L. (2003). *Quality in qualitative evaluation: A framework for assessing research evidence*. Government Chief Social Researcher's Office, Prime Minister's strategy Unit, London. Retrieved from www.strategy.gov. uk on 29 January 2013.

Stein, A. (2010). Sex, truths, and audiotape: Anonymity and the ethics of public exposure in ethnography. *Journal of Contemporary Ethnography, 39*(5), 554–568.

Stewart, K. & Williams, M. (2005). Researching online populations: The use of online focus groups for social research. *Qualitative Research, 5*(4), 395–416.

Stratton, P. (2010). *The evidence base of systematic family and couples therapies*. London: The Association for Family Therapy & Systemic Practice.

Tapscott, D. & Williams, A. (2008). *Wikinomics: How mass collaboration changes everything*. New York: Portfolio.

Tates, K. & Meeuwesen, L. (2000). Let mum have her say: Turn-taking in doctor-parent-child communication. *Patient Education and Counseling, 40*, 151–162.

Taylor, H., Stuttaford, M., Broad, B. & Vostanis, P. (2006). 'Why a roof is not enough': The characteristics of young homeless people referred to a designated mental health service. *Journal of Mental Health, 15*(4), 491–501.

Teijlingen (van), E., Rennie, A. M., Hundley, V. & Graham, W. (2001). The importance of conducting and reporting pilot studies: The example of the Scottish births survey. *Journal of Advanced Nursing, 34*(3), 289–295.

Ten Have, P. (2002). Ontology or methodology? Comments on Speer's 'natural' and 'contrived' data: A sustainable distinction? *Discourse Studies, 4*(4), 527–530.

Terry, W., Olson, G., Ravenscroft, P., Wilss, L. & Boulton-Lewis, G. (2006). Hospice patients' views on research in palliative care. *Internal Medicine Journal, 36*, 406–413.

Testa, A. & Coleman, L. (2006). Accessing research participants in schools: A case study of UK adolescent sexual health survey. *Health Education Research, 21*(4), 518–526.

Themessl-Huber, M., Humphris, G., Dowell, J., Macgillivray, S., Rushmer, R. & Williams, B. (2008). Audio-visual recording of patient-GP consultations for research purposes: A literature review on recruiting rates and strategies. *Patient Education and Counseling, 71*, 157–168.

Thomas, N. & O'Kane, C. (1998). The ethics of participatory research with children. *Children and Society, 12*, 336–348.

Thompson, D., Kirkman, S., Watson, R. & Stewart, S. (2005). Improving research supervision in nursing. *Nurse Education Today, 25*, 283–290.

Thorne, S. (2000). Data analysis in qualitative research. *Evidence Based Nursing, 3*, 68–70.

Thorne, S. (2009). The role of qualitative research within an evidence-based context: Can metasynthesis be the answer? *International journal of Nursing Studies, 46*, 569–575.

Tilley, S. (2003). Transcription work: Learning through coparticipation in research practices. *Qualitative Studies in Education, 16*(6), 835–851.

Tilley, S. & Powick, K. (2002). Distanced data: Transcribing other people's research tapes. *Canadian Journal of Education, 27*(2/3), 291–310.

Tishler, C. (2011). Pediatric drug-trial recruitment: Enticement without coercion. *Pediatrics, 127*(5), 949–954.

Trivedi, P. & Wykes, T. (2002). From passive subjects to equal partners: Qualitative review of user involvement in research. *British Journal of Psychiatry, 181*, 468–472.

Tuckett, A. (2004). Part 1: Qualitative research sampling – the very real complexities. *Nurse Researcher, 12*(1), 47–61.

Tufte, B. (2006). Tweens as consumers – with focus on girls' and boys' internet use. *Child and Teen Consumption, 53,* 1–18.

Unger, J., Kipke, M., Simon, T., Montomery, S. & Johnson, C. (1997). Homeless youths and young adults in Los Angeles: Prevalence of mental health problems and the relationship between mental health and substance abuse disorders. *American Journal of Community Psychology, 25,* 371–394.

Valke, M., De Wever, B., Van Keer, H. & Schellens, T. (2011). Long-term study of safe internet use of young children. *Computers and Education, 57,* 1292–1305.

Waddell, C. & Godderis, R. (2005). Rethinking evidence-based practice for children's mental health. *Evidence Based Mental Health, 8,* 60–62.

Waller, T. & Bitou, A. (2011). Research with children: Three challenges for participatory research in early childhood. *European Early Childhood Education Research Journal, 19*(1), 5–20.

Warming, H. (2011). Getting under their skins? Accessing young children's perspectives through ethnographic fieldwork. *Childhood, 18*(1), 39–53.

Wartella, E. & Jennings, N. (2000). Children and computers: New technology-old concerns. *The Future of Children, 10*(2), 31–43.

Watson, R. (1997). Ethnomethodology and textual analysis. In D. Silverman (ed.), *Qualitative research: Theory, method and practice* (pp. 80–98). London: Sage.

White, P. (2009). *Developing research questions: A guide for social scientists.* Hampshire: Palgrave Macmillan.

Widdowson, H. G. (2004). *Text, context, pretext: Critical studies in discourse analysis.* Oxford: Blackwell.

Wilkinson, M. & Moore, A. (1997). Inducement to research. *Bioethics, 11*(5), 373–389.

Wilkinson, S., Joffe, H. & Yardley, L. (2004). Qualitative data collection: Interviews and focus groups. In D. Marks & L. Yardley (eds), *Research methods for clinical and health psychology* (pp. 38–55). London: Sage.

Williamson, E., Goodenough, T., Kent, J. & Ashcroft, R. (2005). Conducting research with children: The limits of confidentiality and child protection protocols. *Children and Society, 19,* 397–409.

Willig, C. (2001). *Introducing qualitative research: Adventures in theory and method.* Buckingham: Open University Press.

Willmott, A., (2010). Involving children: How to do it. In S. Redsell & A. Hastings (eds), *Listening to children and young people in healthcare consultations* (pp. 45–55). Oxon: Radcliffe Publishing.

Wilson, J. & Hunter, D. (2010). Research exceptionalism. *The American Journal of Bioethics, 10*(8), 45–54.

Wilson, C. & Powell, M. (2001). *A Guide to interviewing children: Essential skills for counsellors, police, lawyers and social workers.* Sydney: Allen and Unwin.

Wind, G. (2008). Negotiated interactive observation: Doing fieldwork in hospital settings. *Anthropology and Medicine, 15*(2), 79–89.

Wong, P-H. J. & Poon, K-L. M. (2010). Bringing translation out of the shadows: Translation as an issue of methodological significance in cross-cultural qualitative research. *Journal of Transcultural Nursing, 21*(2), 151–158.

Woodhead, M. & Faulkner, D. (2000). Subjects, objects or participants? Dilemmas of psychological research with children. In P. Christensen & A. James (eds), *Research with children: Perspectives and practices* (pp. 9–35). London: Falmer Press.

Wooffitt, R. (2005). *Conversation analysis and discourse analysis: A comparative and critical introduction.* London: Sage.

Wooffitt, R. & Widdicombe, S. (2006). Interaction in interviews. In P. Drew, G. Raymond & D. Weinberg (eds), *Talk and interaction in social research methods* (pp. 29–49). London: Sage.

World Health Organization. (2011). *Mental health: A state of well-being.* Retrieved from www.who.int/features/factfiles/mental_health/en/ on 18 January 2012.

Wright, K., (2005). Researching internet-based populations: Advantages and disadvantages of online survey research, online questionnaire authoring software packages, and web survey services. *Journal of Computer-Mediated Communication, 10*(3), article 11. Retrieved from http//jcmc.indiana.edu/vol10/issue3/wright.html on 25 March 2013.

Yip, K-S., (2006). Self-reflective practice: A note of caution. *British Journal of Social Work, 36,* 777–788.

Zimmer, M. (2010). 'But the data is already public': On the ethics of research in Facebook. *Ethics and Information Technology, 12,* 313–325.

INDEX